reflex®
Tomorrow's Nutrition Today™

GUIDE TO
BODY
TONING

Welcome to the *Women's Fitness Guide to Body Toning*, which is dedicated to helping you achieve a firm and lean figure. If you want to lose some weight, you'll find plenty of advice in our cardio section, but the main emphasis in this book is to help you sculpt
and tone your body, using safe exercises that really work.

We know that motivation is a key ingredient of a successful exercise routine, so we've devoted a whole chapter to it, starting on page 15. If you find you can't stick to a regular exercise routine, or you're struggling to get started, you'll find lots of expert tips to help you on your way.

This book has everything you need to enjoy getting fit, toned and fabulous!

Joanna

Editor Joanna Knight
Art Director Matt Reynolds
Editorial Assistant Amanda Khouv
Contributors Jeff Archer, Penny Carroll, Anita Ellis, Dave Fletcher, Anne-Marie Lategan, Louise Pyne
Photography Eddie MacDonald; Danny Bird; Shutterstock
Cover model Anel, MOT Models, www.motmodel.com
Model Emily Crompton and Kate Imogen, both W Athletic, www.wathletic.com

Digital Production Manager Nicky Baker
Management MagBook
Publisher Dharmesh Mistry
Operations Director Robin Ryan
Advertising Manager Katie Wood
MD of Advertising Julian Lloyd-Evans
Newstrade Director David Barker
Chief Operating Officer Brett Reynolds
Group Finance Director Ian Leggett
Chief Executive James Tye
Chairman Felix Dennis

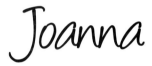

The MagBook brand is a trademark of Dennis Publishing Ltd. 30 Cleveland St, London W1T 4JD. Company registered in England. All material © Dennis Publishing Ltd, licensed by Felden 2012, and may not be reproduced in whole or part without the consent of the publishers. *Guide To Body Toning* ISBN 1781060223.

Clothing credits
Cover
Crop top, £36, Tonic at www.krsc.co.uk
Shorts, £14, www.jdsports.co.uk

Boxing Workout
All sports bra, £28, www.sweatybetty.com
Leggings, £25, www.nikestore.com
Nike Free TR Twist SL trainers, £70, www.nikestore.com

Main Workout
Dream Big Bra, £32,
www.yamarama.com
I Like Short shorts, £35, www.yamarama.com
Nike Air Span+6 trainers, £68.60, www.nikestore.com

Fat Burning Workout
Crop top, £30, www.adidas.com
Curve shorts, £34, www.noballs.co.uk
Nike Lunarglide +3 trainers, £85, www.nikestore.com

Equipment
All from Physical Company, www.physicalcompany.co.uk
Mats from Manuka Life, www.manukalife.co.uk

Licensing & Syndication
To license this product, please contact Carlotta Serantoni on +44 (0) 20 7907 6550 or email carlotta_serantoni@dennis.co.uk
To syndicate content from this product, please contact Anj Dosaj Halai on +44 (0) 20 7907 6132 or email anj_dosaj-halai@dennis.co.uk

Liability
While every care was taken during the production of this MagBook, the publishers cannot be held responsible for the accuracy of the information or any consequence arising from it. Dennis Publishing takes no responsibility for the companies advertising in this MagBook. The paper used within this MagBook is produced from sustainable fibre, manufactured by mills with a valid chain of custody. Printed at BGPrint Ltd.

Always check with your GP before commencing an exercise programme, especially if you have been inactive for a long period of time. Those with a history of high blood pressure or heart disease should obtain medical clearance before undertaking any activity.

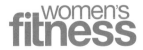

contents

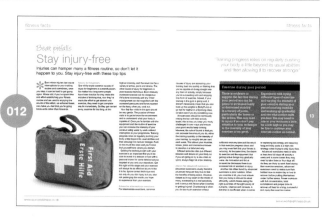

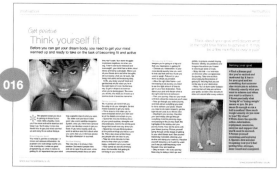

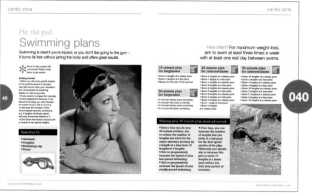

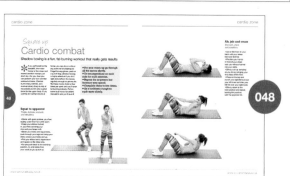

Cardio

6

Contents

Workouts

Brand new fat-loss special

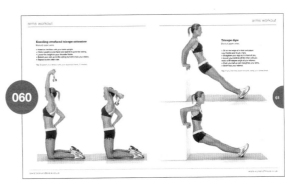

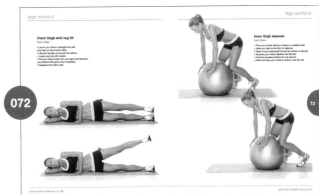

7

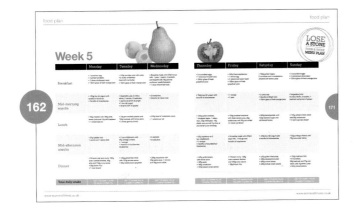

Nutrition

Brand new fat-loss special

The golden rules
Fitness questions

Everything you need to know about exercise intensity and frequency and getting the most from your fitness plan

Many people who exercise regularly don't always get the results they want – usually because they are stuck in a rut with their training and following an old programme that doesn't challenge them any more. It could also be because they are counteracting their hard work by consuming extra calories that they aren't burning off, that they aren't training as regularly as they need to be, or even that they aren't working hard enough when they do exercise.

There's nothing more demoralising than feeling like you are doing everything you should be doing, only to find you're not losing weight or toning up. Follow our guidelines here to ensure that every moment you spend exercising will count.

Exercise training zones

Moderate Aerobic Zone
50-60 per cent of maximum heart rate (MHR). This is mainly for looking after your health and is a moderate intensity, ideal for beginners or those who are looking for a gentle workout.

Weight Management Zone
60-70 per cent of MHR. This is often called the 'fat burning zone'. This intensity is moderate enough to sustain for long periods of time, which means that you can use fat as the main source of energy, but also means you need to exercise for longer periods of time, i.e. 40 minutes upwards.

Aerobic Fitness Zone
70-80 per cent of MHR. This is mainly to improve your stamina. It is called the 'aerobic training zone' and means you are working at a higher intensity, which is more challenging and will increase your fitness.

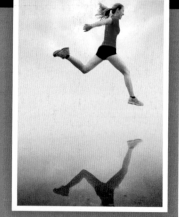

How often should I exercise?
If your main aim is to stay healthy, the American College of Sports Medicine recommends moderate-intensity cardio of 30 minutes a day, five days a week, or vigorous, intense cardio 20 minutes a day, three days a week, plus eight to ten strength-training exercises (such as press-ups, BodyPump or lifting weights). Aim for eight to 12 repetitions of each exercise twice a week. Moderate-intensity physical activity means working hard enough to raise your heart rate and break a sweat, yet still being able to carry on a conversation with relative ease.

How often should I exercise for weight-loss?
Aim for 30 minutes of high-intensity or 45 minutes of moderate-intensity cardio exercise five times a week, e.g. running, jogging, power-walking or cycling, or try exercise classes, e.g. circuit training, kickboxing or aerobics.

8

'Interval training is the best way to maximise results, which means changing your intensity during your workout'

How hard should I work during my cardio sessions?

Interval training is the best way to maximise your results. This means that you have to change the intensity during your workout between low intensity (training at about 50 per cent of your maximum heart rate), moderate (training at about 70 per cent of your MHR), and high (training at about 80 per cent of your MHR).

To determine your maximum heart rate (MHR) and your training intensity, use the following formulas:

Maximum heart rate = 206 – 88% age
For example a 30-year-old will have a maximum heart rate of 88% of 30 years = 26.4
206 – 26.4 = 179.6, or 180bpm

Fitter individuals use: 205 – 50% age
For example a fitter 30-year-old will have a maximum heart rate of 50% of 30 years = 15
205 – 15 = 190bpm

Alternating between low, moderate and high intensities allows you to work hard for short periods of time, as this will increase your calorie usage. As a beginner, alternate your intensity between low (50 per cent of MHR) and moderate (70 per cent of MHR) intensity. As your fitness levels improve, increase your sprint intensity to your high-intensity heart rate (80 per cent of MHR).

Activity calorie guide

Activity	Calories used in 30 minutes
Walking, 2 mph, slow pace	85
Walking, 3 mph, moderate pace	118
Walking, 3-5 mph, uphill	204
Walking, 4 mph, brisk pace	134
Running, 5 mph (12-min mile)	271
Running, 6 mph (10-min mile)	340
Running, 7 mph (8.5-min mile)	389
Running, 8 mph (7.5-min mile)	459
Running, 9 mph (6.5-min mile)	510
Cycling, 10-12 mph	204
Cycling, 12-14 mph	271
Cycling, 14-16 mph	340
Dancing – ballet, modern, twist	204
Aerobics, low impact	169
Aerobics, high impact	238
Rope jumping, moderate effort	340
Skiing, downhill, light effort	169
Skiing, downhill, moderate effort	204
Skiing, downhill, vigorous effort	271
Swimming, moderate effort	271
Swimming, vigorous effort	340

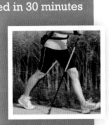
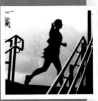
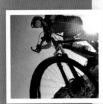
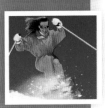

9

What type of cardio exercise is best?
Exercise that makes use of large muscle groups, such as running, cycling or swimming, is best. It takes about six weeks for your body to adapt to a routine, so after that, either change the frequency you exercise, the intensity of your exercise, the time you exercise for, or the type of exercise.

Should I split up my sessions?
If time isn't an issue, you may find that you can have a better cardio session if you focus on it solely in one session, and the same applies with weights. However, if you are simply looking to burn some calories and tone up, but you're short of time, you should be able to do both weights and cardio in one session. If you do weights first, you could do one set on a certain machine and then move on to another without stopping and then repeat the circuit.

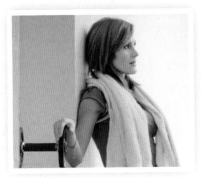

Exercising with asthma

You should be able to do any exercise, providing your asthma is controlled. Activities like hiking or skiing at high altitudes or in cold weather can cause problems, so consult your doctor before attempting this kind of exercise. Swimming, circuit classes, team sports and yoga are all good examples of physical activities to try. Long-distance running and cycling can cause asthma attacks, but many people can jog or run marathons without problems.

- Always carry your inhaler with you when you exercise.
- Start slowly and build your fitness levels gradually.
- Use your inhaler before exercise if your asthma is exercise induced.

- Never train alone outside.
- If you are training in a group, inform the instructor about your asthma.
- Warm up and cool down for at least ten minutes.
- Train in your comfort zone – don't push yourself too hard.
- Exercising in moist, hot air is less likely to irritate your airways compared to cold, dry conditions.
- Avoid exercising outdoors if the pollen levels are particularly high.
- Don't exercise if you have a cold or chest infection.

Asthma UK gives help and advice on how to live with asthma: call 08456 038 143 or visit www.asthma.org.uk

Sound smart!
Exercise speak

Know your reps from your sets and your flexibility
from your motor skills with our 'gym speak' guide

 Baffled by words you've heard
in the gym? Our guide will
clear up the confusion…

Anaerobic exercise
High-intensity exercise that burns
glycogen for energy, instead of
oxygen. Anaerobic exercise creates a
temporary oxygen deficit by consuming
more oxygen than the body can
supply. Example: weight-lifting.

Burn
The sensation in a muscle when
it has been worked intensely.
It is caused by a build-up
of waste products and microscopic
muscle tears during exercise.

Cardiovascular exercise
Activity in which the body is able
to supply adequate oxygen to the
working muscles, for a period of
time. Examples: running or cycling.

Exercise intensity
The amount of force or energy you
expend during a workout, i.e. how
hard you work during exercise.

Fat-burning zone
Used during cardiovascular exercise

and refers to the exercise intensity
at which the body uses stored fat
for energy. At approximately 60 to
70 per cent of your maximum
heart rate, about 85 per
cent of calories burned in
this zone are fats, five per
cent are proteins and ten
per cent are carbohydrates.

Flexibility
Range of movement
(ROM) in a joint or group
of joints. Good flexibility
refers to an advanced
degree of suppleness in
the joints and muscles.

Motor skills
A movement that involves
muscle groups and the
function of the brain
working in unison.
This includes
practically all forms
of movement,
including
walking, kicking,
jumping,
climbing stairs and
working out. It also
refers to balance.

Muscular endurance
The ability of a muscle to produce
force continually over a period of
time. Example: circuit training.

Muscular strength
The ability of a muscle to
produce maximum force,
e.g. using weights.

Reps
A shortening of
repetitions, this means
one complete
movement of
an exercise.

Sets
These are the fixed
number of repetitions,
e.g. ten repetitions
may comprise one set.

Target heart rate
The speed at which you
keep your heartbeat during
aerobic exercise. Find
your target heart rate by
multiplying your maximum
heart rate by 0.7 (for 70
per cent) and by 0.8
(for 80 per cent).

11

Beat pitfalls
Stay injury-free

Injuries can hamper many a fitness routine, so don't let it happen to you. Stay injury-free with these top tips

Even minor injuries can cause interruptions to your training routine and sometimes, once you stop, it can be hard to get going again. Worse still, if you've spent time and effort establishing your fitness routine and are used to enjoying the results of this effort, an enforced break can make you feel that you're going backwards rather than forwards.

Advice for beginners
One of the most common causes of injury for beginners is overenthusiasm. No matter how long some people have been inactive for they make the mistake of thinking that, now they've made the effort to get started with exercise, they need to get complete results immediately. So they get carried away, exercise for too long, at too high an intensity, and the result can be a variety of aches, pains and strains. The other cause of injury for beginners is poor exercise technique. Even relatively moderate exercise can be dangerous if it's done incorrectly and any minor misalignment can be magnified with the increased pressures and forces exerted on the body when you work out.

Your first few visits to the gym should be very gentle. The purpose of these visits is to get to know the environment and to understand what your body is capable of. Once you're familiar with the equipment and the routine of exercise you can increase the intensity of your workout safely week by week without interruption to your programme. Training progress relies on regularly pushing your body a little beyond its usual abilities and then allowing it to recover stronger. Push on too much too soon and you'll soon find yourself back where you started.

Getting the technique right with your exercise is so important that you'd be wise to invest in a session or two with a personal trainer for some detailed advice targeted at you and your objectives. Get this right at this stage and your exercise will always be as effective as you'd like it to be. Ignore correct technique and not only do you risk injury, but you also risk prolonging the results you hope to experience from your exercise.

Advice for intermediate exercisers
For intermediate exercisers, common

12

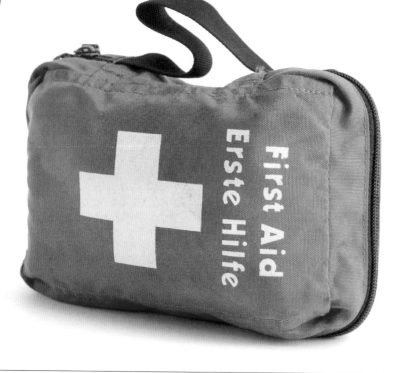

'Training progress relies on regularly pushing your body a little beyond its usual abilities and then allowing it to recover stronger'

causes of injury are increasing your training load too quickly or thinking that you're capable of diving straight into any form of activity, simply because you're succeeding with and enjoying one form of exercise. Indeed, if your training in the gym is going well, it doesn't necessarily mean that you can load up the weights in BodyPump or go hell for leather in a Spinning class, so take care if you try something new.

All exercisers should be continually raising the bar with their activity levels; this is how you keep your body challenged in new ways and ensure your good results keep coming. However, the rule of thumb is that you can increase the amount you do, either the training quantity or the intensity of your training, by roughly ten per cent each week. This allows your muscles, bones, joints and connective tissues to develop in a balanced way.

Different activities also put different stresses and strains on your body so if you are going to try a new class or sport, always begin at a low intensity.

Advice for advanced exercisers

Advanced exercisers usually become advanced because they love to feel the benefits of being active. However, distant as it may seem in the minds of many, overtraining is a real possibility and a serious risk factor when it comes to getting injured. Overtraining is when you do too much exercise without

Exercise during your period

There is evidence to support the fact that during your period you can be prone to increased laxity or decreased stability in a variety of joints, particularly the knees or the ankles. This may lead to injury if you don't pay attention to your technique or the intensity of your exercise is too great.

Experiment with trying different types of exercise and varying the intensity of your exercise during your period (starting carefully and working up gradually) and see what routine suits you best. You may need to rein in your workouts a little for a few days or you may be fine to continue your exercise routine as normal.

13

sufficient recovery time and the result is that exercise progress slows and you may even feel that your fitness is reducing. At the same time, the desire to exercise and the enjoyment that getting active brings may gradually wane. As motivation and focus on exercise decreases there is an increased risk of accident or injury.

Another risk often faced by advanced exercisers is poor nutrition. When you exercise a lot, you must ensure that your body is allowed to refuel efficiently, which means eating the right quantities of the right variety of nutrients, vitamins and minerals. A diet that is insufficient when it comes

to replacing lost energy and repairing fatigued body parts is a high-risk strategy when trying to stay injury-free.

Advanced exercisers need to take at least two full days off activity a week and in some cases they may need to take three or four days off. As they are likely to work hard during their exercise sessions, advanced exercisers need to make sure their bodies have an entire day or two to recover before putting themselves under further stress. Fewer workouts with full concentration, total commitment and proper time to recover will lead to a long, successful and injury-free exercise career.

Banish the bounce

Protect your bust

Keep your breasts firm and prevent sagging with our guide to choosing the right sports bra for you and your chosen activity

Struggling to find a decent sports bra? Or do you suffer from breast pain when you work out? You are not alone. According to a recent report, around three in five women suffer from breast pain during exercise, because they are wearing the wrong bra. Some bras may stop breasts from bouncing up and down during sport, but don't prevent them from moving from side to side. Researchers examined women with cup sizes from A to JJ and found that even small-breasted women could suffer discomfort when exercising. The report concluded that many women did not wear the correct support and often make the mistake of choosing a large bra size with too small a cup, rather than vice versa.

The right bra
A correctly fitting sports bra is essential for providing support when jogging, and it also improves posture. The Cooper's ligament, which is a band of elastic tissue that stops your breasts from drooping, starts to stretch as you get older and pulls the breasts down. If you don't support your breasts, you will speed up this process and they will begin to sag in time.

Don't be embarrassed
If you have a large bust, you may feel self-conscious, but remember that other women may be envious, so be proud of your assets. A sports bra will reduce the bounce, but there may still be some movement, so wear a loose top or T-shirt over it to spare your blushes. If you are shy of stripping off in the gym changing rooms, choose a gym that provides a cubicle where you can get changed privately.

Diet and exercise
As the bust is made up of fatty tissue and not muscle, by reducing your calorie intake and increasing your exercise levels, you will certainly lose weight and your bust size will

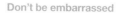

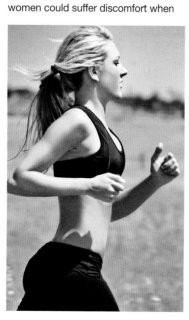

Choosing a sports bra

■ Get your bust measured first so that you know your exact size.
■ Choose the right impact level for your sport.
■ Change your bra if you lose or gain weight, as your bust size will change.

decrease. But in order to keep your breasts from sagging, you should also exercise. You can't actually firm up the breasts, given that they are fatty tissue, but you can aim to give the impression they are firm by training the chest muscles that surround the breasts. The best exercise is the simple press-up. You can stay on your knees at first and slowly build up the repetitions to take your weight on your arms and toes.

Breast reduction
A correctly fitting sports bra will keep you well-supported and also give you the confidence to work out. Choose a high-impact bra if you are going to be running or doing sports that involve bursts of running or jumping. Remember to change your bra regularly too, just like your trainers!

14

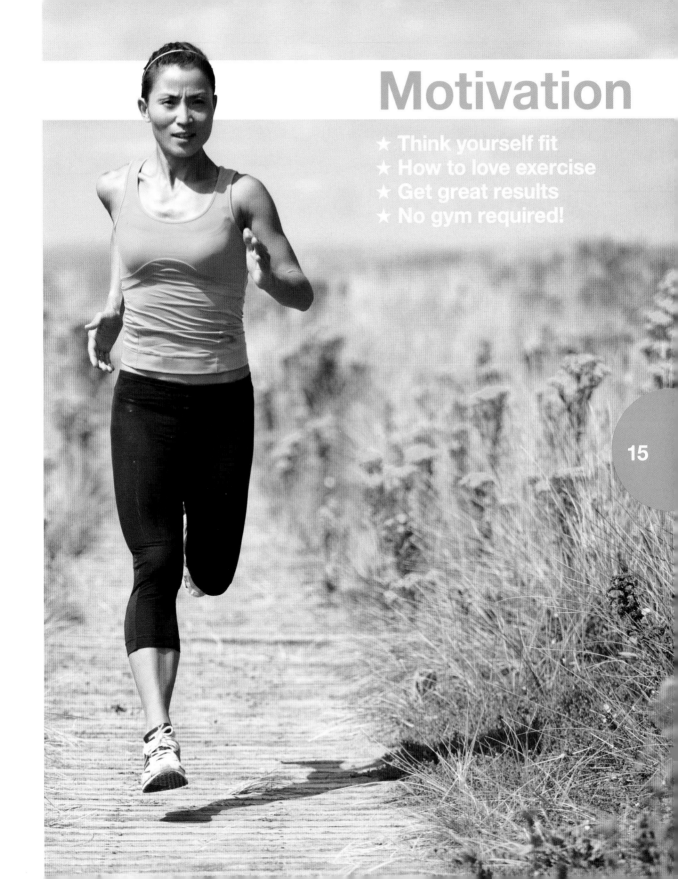

Motivation

★ Think yourself fit
★ How to love exercise
★ Get great results
★ No gym required!

15

Get positive

Think yourself fit

Before you can get your dream body, you need to get your mind warmed up and ready to take on the task of becoming fit and active

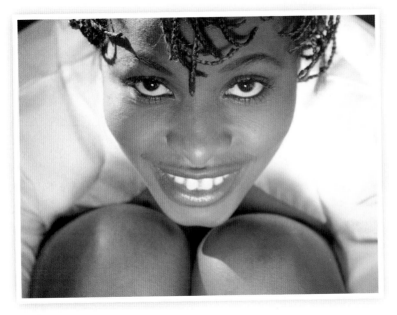

The greatest asset you have to getting in shape is your mind. With a healthy mind, you'll be more inclined to exercise and keep it up. You'll enjoy it more too. Here's how to get your mind warmed up and ready for an active lifestyle.

Mastering your mind
Your mind is just like a computer – it stores and retrieves information. Its purpose is to work things out for you. Like a computer, it relies on good programming, so when it comes to getting fit, it's important that your mind has a specific idea of what you want.

So, make sure you have a clear goal. Like a car's satellite-navigation system, once your mind has a precise goal it can develop a route to get you there. If you know exactly what you want to achieve and think about what you want, then your mind can access the right information to succeed.

Positive thinking
The next step is to always think positive. Successful people think and act on what they do want, while unsuccessful people focus on what

they don't want. Your mind struggles to process negatives, so when you say, 'I don't want to be stressed and overweight', your mind has to think about stress and being overweight. Make sure all your fitness aims and other thoughts set out exactly what you do want, like being motivated and exercising daily.

In life, you enjoy yourself most and get the best results when you're in the right frame of mind. So the best way to get in shape is to exercise when you're feeling good. The more you do this, the more you'll build up a positive bank of exercise memories.

Fitness success
Your success will come from you focusing on all your strengths. Do this mental exercise to get you ready.
■ Think about a time when you've been energised and at your best and let all the details come back to you.
■ Spend ten minutes thinking about all your good qualities, strengths and characteristics. Add to this all the good things that loved ones say about you.
■ Spend ten minutes thinking about all the positive things you have in your life. Think also about all the things and people who are dear to you.
■ Take ten more minutes to think about a time when you've been happy, confident and at your best.
■ Now spend ten minutes thinking about the benefits that getting fit will bring to your whole life.

'Think about your goal and decide what is the right time frame to achieve it. It may be a few months or over a year'

Your journey to fitness

Imagine you're going on a trip and that your destination is getting fit!

■ Choose your destination. In your mind decide exactly how you want to look and feel and how much you want to weigh. Picture it in your mind as clearly as possible.

■ Allow the right time frame – just like making a car journey you need to set the right amount of time to get to your final destination. Think about your goal and decide what is the right time frame to achieve it.

■ Plan your journey. Map out your route and think about the resources you'll need.

■ Now go through your entire journey and think about everything you need to do to achieve your goals. Maybe you need to do some research, get the right kit and work out a fitness plan.

■ Daydream your journey. Visualise your last holiday and go through everything from the planning stage and packing to the journey itself, the highlights of the holiday and your journey home. Now do the same with your fitness journey. Picture yourself going through all the stages of getting to your ideal fitness level. See yourself becoming motivated, planning your routine and doing your workout. Visualise yourself enjoying it, and week by week you'll see yourself becoming more focused, fitter and healthier.

■ Stay on track – like every journey there may be delays, hold-ups and pitfalls, so picture yourself staying focused. Identify any problems and imagine the actions you'll need to take to get back on track.

■ Enjoy the ride – our best trips are the ones when we appreciate the journey. Take time to think about enjoying the process of getting fit, knowing that you are on the way to your destination.

■ Relax. You've done some fantastic exercise that will help you achieve your goals, so take a few minutes to relax and unwind after every workout.

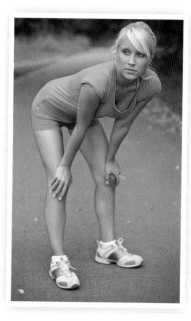

Setting your goal

■ Find a fitness goal that you're excited and motivated by. It has to be your goal and not something that someone else wants you to achieve.

■ Identify exactly what you want to achieve and when you want to achieve it.

■ Know precisely what 'being fit' or 'losing weight' means to you. Do you mean fit enough to run a half marathon? How much weight exactly do you want to lose? By when?

■ Write down the specific action, information, equipment, resources, exercise and support that you'll need to succeed.

■ Picture yourself exercising and enjoying it. Spend a few minutes imagining how you'll feel getting fitter, stronger, more toned and energised.

17

Up the fun factor
How to love exercise

Don't quit your exercise routine through boredom. It's easy to maintain an exercise plan when you know how to make it fun

Ask almost anyone if they would like to get fitter, feel better, improve their body tone and increase their energy levels, and the answer would be a resounding 'yes'. So why do many people struggle to reach their objectives? Here are some of the most common reasons why exercise can be difficult to fit into a regular routine, along with some suggestions of ways to overcome common objections to exercising that we all have at one time or another...

I try to exercise but I find it boring. What can I do?

Exercise is often deemed to be boring when you think about going to the gym for a long time or stepping out for a lengthy walk or run. The thought that your exercise routine, along with all the preparation and travel that go with it, might not be over for a couple of hours can feel like just too much to bear. The idea of spending 20 to 30 minutes or more on a particular cardio machine, or running through the same exercise programme or class, can also fill you with despair.

Instead, complete your exercise in short, intensive bursts. We're all pushed for time and our attention span can be short given our other commitments, so aim to get the most benefit from your workout in the shortest possible time.
- Spend only five or ten minutes on any CV machine, but work hard for the entire duration of that time.
- Set yourself objectives like 'I must cover 5K in the shortest possible time' or 'I'll aim to do the majority of this workout on one level higher than last time'. These short, sharp bursts of activity will ensure that your mind doesn't begin to wander.
- Don't scrimp on the quality of your exercise. Make sure you're always using good posture and always use safe techniques.
- Keep your exercise routine fresh. Try a variety of exercises in the gym or take some classes as part of your schedule. Exercise outdoors in good weather. Make every week of your exercise programme different, so there's no reason to get bored.

I find exercise uncomfortable, it's just too strenuous. What can I do?

Exercising is never going to feel as comfortable as sitting on the sofa or being out with your friends – basically, inhabiting life in the comfort zone. But just how comfortable is your so-called 'comfort zone'? You're probably very hard on yourself when you don't exercise and this criticism can be quite painful in its own way, so find a level of exercise or some activities or team sports that provide you with enough of a workout for you to see and feel fitness improvements.
- Make sure you have the correct clothing for your exercise. If it's too loose, you'll get distracted. If it's too tight, you'll feel constricted.
- You also need to ensure you have the right footwear for your chosen activity.
- Your exercise environment should be cool and airy. If you get too hot, you'll soon start to feel uncomfortable.
- Begin gently and increase your intensity slowly over time. This will

Easy ways to stay motivated

- **Make exercise social. Find a class with a friend that you both enjoy and make it quality time you spend together.**
- **Listen to upbeat music while you exercise.**
- **Try short workouts when time is precious. 20 minutes of cardio at a slightly higher intensity will still count.**
- **Vary your workouts to keep your enthusiasm up.**

18

'Schedule your workouts in advance and aim to exercise every two to three days. Plan what you will do on recovery days'

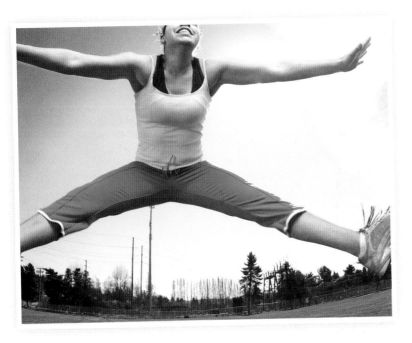

■ For best results, plan workouts in advance and aim to exercise every two to three days. An exercise programme that fits into your overall schedule is one that you will stick with.
■ Plan what you will do on your rest and recovery days, so that you use your time well, fulfil work duties, enjoy your social time, and keep exercise time free from any distractions.

19

I've tried exercising before and it didn't work, so why should I bother this time? What can I do differently?
If exercise hasn't worked for you in the past, then you just haven't found the right exercise programme that works for you yet. Be positive; the more programmes you've tried, the more options you've eliminated, so the closer you are now to finding the correct routine.
■ Decide right now that this time, exercise will work for you.
■ Think about what 'working' means to you. What specific results are you looking for? When do you want to see those results? What do you need to do to ensure you get those results? How important is it to you? Are you willing to make this a priority?
■ Once you have answered these questions, experiment with different types of exercise, workout patterns, different intensities and durations with your workouts, and keep modifying until you get the results you want.

ensure that you never become too uncomfortable during your workout.
■ Plan rest periods into your workout.
■ Try something that doesn't feel like exercise. Cycling on a sunny day or swimming with the family will burn calories and you'll enjoy yourself.

I start well but soon give up, as I often find there's something better to do! What can I do?
Finding creative ways to distract yourself from your exercise programme could be an Olympic sport in itself!

When it's time to get to the gym, somehow anything seems more exciting – even tidying up the kitchen!
Fitness programmes usually begin with good intentions, but these can wane if results are not fast enough, and it's at this point that we can become easily distracted. If your programme produces results that you are pleased with in a short space of time, you are unlikely to waver off-track. You'll be so excited about how great you feel, you'll be counting down to each workout to ensure the results still keep coming.

Fail-proof plan
Get great results

To help you get the most from your workouts every time you hit the gym, we provide the answers to some common exercise dilemmas

Whether it's reaching a fitness plateau, finding your classes repetitive or simply being bored by the treadmill, you may encounter a variety of dilemmas when it comes to exercise. Here are some common issues that crop up, along with solutions to overcome them.

Dilemma 1

I don't seem to be getting any fitter on the cardio machines and I'm not getting any stronger on the weights. What am I doing wrong?

Chances are, you've been doing the same routine for too long and it simply doesn't challenge you enough.
■ Try shortening your workouts on the cardio machines, but make them more intense. Walk, run, row or cycle as far as you can in only ten minutes on each machine. Once you've set your benchmark distances, aim to improve on these each time you work out.
■ For strength training, push yourself to experiment with heavier weights and vary the exercises you do. Provided you can still complete 15-20 reps with the weights you're using, you won't bulk up.
■ Increase the resistance for all your strength-training exercises. Challenge yourself by using a heavier weight in order to make faster progress.

Dilemma 2

My partner wants us to train together, but he wants to get big muscles and I want to lose weight. Can we train together?
Training with a partner is a great idea, provided you structure your workouts to work for both of you.
■ For the bulk of your workout, you can use the same cardio and strength training machines, even though you will both have different objectives.
■ On cardio machines, you should both be working hard for relatively short bursts of activity. When strength training, use lighter weights for longer sets of 15 to 20, or even 25, reps, while your partner can use heavier weights for less reps.
■ Stick together for the exercises using major muscle groups (back and biceps, chest and triceps, shoulders and legs) and then split up for a couple of supplementary exercises. You may wish to do more lower-body exercises, while your partner might like to add a couple of extra upper-body exercises.

Dilemma 3

I get very bored on the cardio machines, but I need to lose weight and burn calories. What can I do?
The answer to 'cardio tedium' is to keep your workouts short and sweet. Avoid steady training, because even

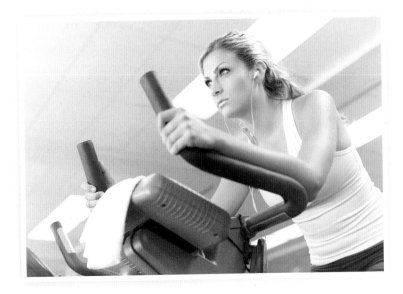

'Walk, run, row or cycle as far as you can in only ten minutes, and aim to improve on your distance each time you work out'

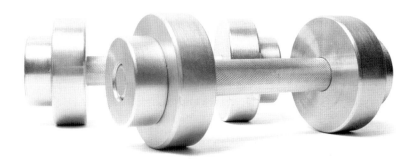

three minutes at the same speed and intensity can seem like a lifetime when you're not in the mood.

■ Use interval training, where you alternate tough bursts of intense activity with bouts of recovery. Push hard for one minute, followed by a minute or so of recovery.

■ Try stepped workouts, where you gradually increase the levels of difficulty from easy through to tough before repeating the sequence.

■ You could also try pyramid training, where you change your level of intensity each minute or so, or you can try a 'two steps forward, one step back' pattern, both of which will make your workout more varied.

Dilemma 4

My mum wants to start working out with me at the gym, but I'm worried because she's not exercised for years. What should I do?

For working out with anyone who hasn't exercised for a long time, follow the same advice:

■ Ask them to check with a doctor that they are OK to exercise and then have them take part in an initial health screening or consultation at the gym.

■ Encourage them to think about what they want out of their gym visits and when they want these results.

■ Then urge them to take advice from gym staff on what type of programme will ensure the desired results.

Dilemma 5

I can only manage to get to my gym twice a week, but I really need to lose a few pounds. What can I do?

If your workout time is limited make sure that the little time you do have in the gym is used wisely.

■ Spend ten minutes on each cardio machine but really work hard.

■ Using the treadmill or the rowing machine can help you to work harder than the step machine or the bike, as they force you to use your whole body rather than just the bottom half.

■ Strength training should be focused on exercises that use many muscles at once, like upper back pull-down, seated rows, squats and lunges. Working different muscle groups by alternating exercises also helps to burn more calories.

■ Try and fit as much activity into your daily and work routine as possible. Practise good posture at all times to look after your spine, and make every journey a fitness burst by swinging your arms, squeezing your bum and speeding along, rather than ambling gently to your next destination.

■ Finally, watch your food quality and portion sizes, and eat for energy and performance, not out of boredom.

Dilemma 6

I hate using weights, but I really need to tone up. What can I do?

If using weights bores you, challenge yourself to try a couple of new exercises every time you visit the gym.

■ Mix up your resistance training by using a combination of free weights, machines, bands and Medicine balls.

■ There are so many options that you almost need never repeat a workout, but if you do get stuck, try going along to a BodyPump class for a great group session that will tone you up and keep you stimulated at the same time.

Work out wherever
No gym required!

If you don't want to go to the gym, you can enjoy home or outdoor workouts and get great results with our guide to indoor and outdoor fitness

You can have an effective workout from the comfort of your living room or bedroom, as long as you warm up, work at the right intensity and stretch afterwards. In fact, the same principles that apply to gym and outdoor exercise apply to working out at home. It's important to exercise regularly enough to get results (ideally four times a week) and ensure you have recovery days in between sessions. Make sure you have enough room around you, especially if you are doing a dance or high-impact aerobics DVD that involves moving the arms outwards. The minimum requirement for a home workout is as much space as you need to stand up in and enough room to extend your arms and legs without hitting any furniture.

By exercising indoors you can ensure you have a range of equipment close by to spice up your routine. Invest in a rope, some resistance bands, a couple of dumbbells, a mat and a stability ball for endless ways to challenge your body. Don't forget to regularly increase the resistance too, as this will help you avoid hitting a plateau.

Spread the effort
If you're at home most of the day, you can spread the effort out. Take an extra lap around the house on the way to the kitchen or go up stairs twice instead of once when you're going to the bedroom. Don't forget to keep your kit handy so you can do a quick set of triceps extensions or shoulder raises whenever you get the urge.

For great motivation when exercising at home, buy yourself a fitness DVD. That way, someone else can plan your exercise routine and when you've

Get the most from home workouts

- Decide when you are going to exercise, write it in your diary and stick to it.
  - Always warm up before you start and stretch at the end of your workout.
  - If you have wooden floors, invest in an exercise mat and wear trainers, not just socks.
  - Wear a sports bra for high-impact exercise.
  - Challenge yourself by maintaining a high intensity for as long as possible, as this will give you the best results.
- Combine your moves. Try shoulder presses and squats in one move, for example.
- Focus on your effort level and results at all times.
- Don't let the TV, music or your mobile distract you.
- Use your environment to be creative with your workout, either with the equipment you use or with the way your programme is structured.
- Remember that four bursts of 15 minutes of activity may be more practical and beneficial to you than aiming for a one-hour workout.

22

'For great motivation at home, buy yourself a fitness DVD. That way, someone else can plan your exercise routine'

mastered the most advanced option on the disc, move on to a new one. Make use of a mirror while you work out too. This will ensure you have good technique and that all your exercises are effective.

Outdoor exercise

If you prefer outdoor exercise, there are plenty of options, especially during the summer when the weather is warmer and the hours of daylight are much longer. Walking or running outdoors are great options, as is cycling. You will usually burn more calories than if you were to run on a treadmill or cycle on a stationary bike in the gym too, as you'll be exercising on uneven surfaces, which will make you work that much harder. If you're used to exercising indoors, taking these pursuits outdoors can seem tough at first because of hilly terrain, so to prepare you could walk or run up and down the stairs a few times to get your legs used to climbing.

Weather conditions

Battling with the weather is something that should also be taken into account if you're used to exercising indoors. If it's windy and rainy outside it can make it feel like you're working much harder than usual, but in fact much of this is actually perceived effort that's experienced by the part of your brain that deals with navigation, staying safe and competing with negative internal dialogue based around the fact that you're battling the elements.

Outdoor exercise safety tips

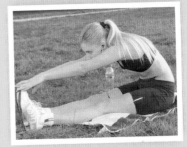

- Take a bottle of water with you and sip it at regular intervals.
- Remember to warm up before you exercise and cool down afterwards.
- Tell someone what your running route is and what time you intend to be home.
- Mix up your routine so that you're not running the same route every time you work out.
- When crossing the roads, cross at proper crossings and make eye contact with a driver before crossing in front of them.
- Run facing oncoming traffic so that you can keep an eye on erratic drivers.
- If you're nervous about exercising outside on your own, invest in a pedometer with a panic alarm. Not only will you be able to monitor calories burned, but it can also be used to fend off would-be muggers.

Cycling, walking or running outdoors forces you to work hard as you contend with hills as well as headwinds. This provides a natural form of sprint or interval training as you'll achieve high-intensity exertion, or possibly even maximum exertion, as you approach the top of a hill, followed by a period of recovery as you reach the flat or descend. It can be hard to push yourself to the limit when you're in the gym, so exercising outside is ideal for pushing yourself to really get the results you want.

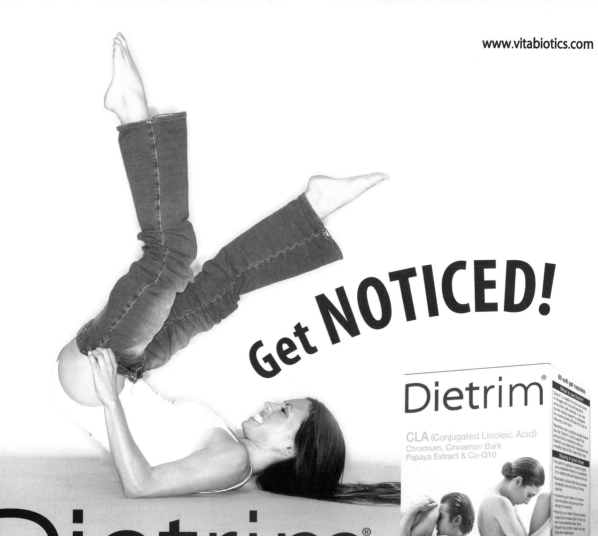

Get NOTICED!

Dietrim®
CAPSULES

Contains
Tonalin CLA®
The Shape Of Things To Come™

Achieving the sort of figure that gets you noticed can be a real challenge.
Dietrim® provides advanced dietary support for when you are working hard to maintain a fit and healthy looking body.
Each capsule contains 26 ingredients for all round health, including biotin and iodine, which <u>play a role in metabolism and in controlling metabollic rate</u>. It also features Tonalin CLA® (Conjugated Linoleic Acid), a scientifically researched ingredient that is derived from the Safflower plant. Dietrim® helps safeguard your nutritional intake if you are on a dieting programme*, or during exercise, without the need for an additional multivitamin.
<u>So let Dietrim® help maintain a healthy you!</u>

Available from Boots, Superdrug, Holland & Barrett, Lloyds pharmacy, Waitrose, pharmacies and health stores or dietrim.co.uk
For more information contact Vitabiotics on 020 8955 2662 or write to us at 1 Apsley Way, London NW2 7HF
Nutritional supplements may benefit those with nutritionally inadequate diets. *This product has not been proven to aid in weight reduction.

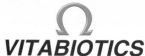

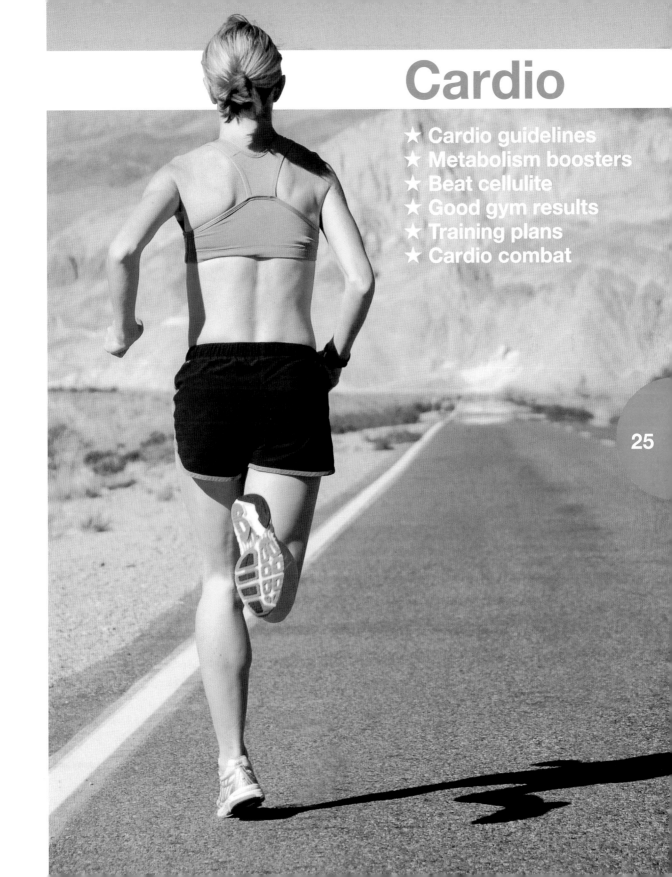

Cardio

★ Cardio guidelines
★ Metabolism boosters
★ Beat cellulite
★ Good gym results
★ Training plans
★ Cardio combat

25

Boost your results

Cardio guidelines

It's one of the best ways to burn fat and lose weight, but how much cardio exercise should you do to see results? Read our guidelines to find out

Cardio exercise is essential if you want to lose weight, but for maximum weight-loss and fitness gains, it's important to consider the following when planning your sessions.

Are you training often enough?
The number of training sessions you do a week is one of the most important things that will determine your progress. According to the American College of Sports Medicine, you should do between three to

five training sessions a week in order to see results. Exercising only twice a week is classified as a maintenance programme, so you will hardly see any results from this.

Are you working hard enough?
The exercise equation is quite simple: the more you put in, the more you'll get out. Using the same speed or weight for more than six weeks will halt your results. This is called a 'plateau'. If you complete an exercise and think 'I don't feel anything' or 'that was

easy', you are probably training in your comfort zone, so you will have to step up the intensity or change the type of exercise you do in order to see results.

How long is your workout?
The time you spend on each exercise will depend on your goals. If you want to be a marathon runner, you have to get the miles in. If you hate your bingo wings, you have to spend more time toning your arms. Without knowing what you want to achieve and your personal time frame, it's impossible to know if you are spending too much or too little time on the different components of your training programme.

When was the last time you changed your programme?
Variety is the key to success! Research has proven that it takes about four to eight weeks for your body to get used to a new exercise. Unless you change the type of exercise, the amount of sets and repetitions or the speed at which you do your exercise, your progression rate will slow down. This is because our bodies are designed to always try to do things easier, quicker and more efficiently.

Do you have a training buddy?
We all like to be part of something and feel like we belong somewhere, and the old saying that we find strength in numbers is very true. Meeting a training buddy at set times will help you get motivated, prevent negative self-talk and

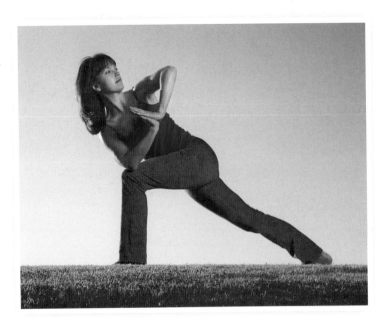

How often? You should do between three to five training sessions a week in order to see results.

stop you thinking of excuses as to why you can't train. According to research, if you do something you enjoy with a friend, you are more likely to achieve your goals than if you train on your own. Surrounding yourself with the type of people you want to be associated with will also improve your self-image and confidence.

Are you overtraining?
This factor is often overlooked. Training

Monitor your intensity

Working out using your heart rate is the most accurate way to determine your intensity, but you can also use the RPE (Rate of Perceived Exertion) scale. This indicates the difficulty level from one to 10, where one is easy and 10 is very hard. Working out at '5', for example, equals about 50 per cent or a low intensity, whereas working out at '7' or '9' represents working out at moderate (70 per cent) or high (90 per cent) intensity.

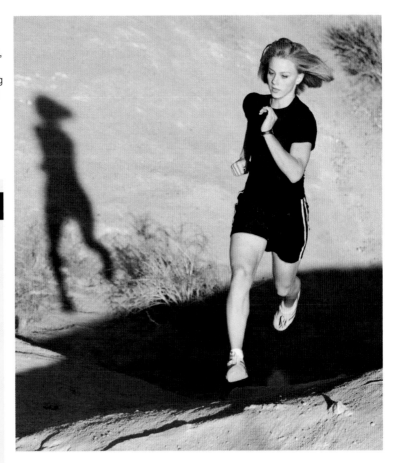

too hard can have the reverse effect on your results. To determine if you are overtraining, ask yourself the following questions. Do you feel more tired training on a Friday than on a Monday? Did you have to reduce your running speed or the amount of weight you lifted over the last few

27

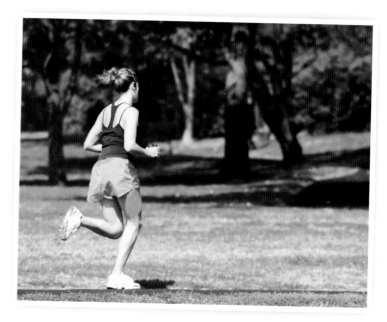

weeks because you just didn't have the energy? Do you wake up feeling drained and exhausted? If you answered yes to any of these questions, you could be doing too much. Stop training for two weeks, rest and get enough sleep in order for your body to recover.

Are you eating the right foods?
Healthy food and plenty of water are very important when you work out regularly. Your body will need carbohydrates like brown rice and pasta for energy, protein such as chicken and eggs to rebuild the muscles and good fats like those found in oily fish to control your immune and hormone systems. Cutting something completely out of your diet can prevent you from losing weight.

Do you know what you are doing?
When you are sick, you go to a doctor. When you struggle to see, you have your eyes tested. If you want to see results and improve your body image, you should consult a fitness professional.

Exercises are very specific and with 640 named muscles in the human body and thousands of unnamed smaller muscles, you should seek professional advice to maximise your potential.

Are you training with injuries?
Never train through an injury because it will slow down your progression. Take time to recover because every time you do something that aggravates the pain, you are re-injuring yourself and prolonging your recovery period.

Do you sleep enough?
We spend about a third of our life asleep. The reason for this is to give our bodies the chance to physically recover (usually between the hours of 10pm and 2am) and to process all the information it has received that day (between 2am and 6am). Lack of sleep can result in loss of strength, coordination, balance and endurance. Prolonged periods of insomnia or sleeplessness can eventually lead to overtraining or injuries.

What time of day should you train?

There is mixed research about what time of the day is the best to train. Some say it's best to train before breakfast on an empty stomach, whereas others say it doesn't matter. The truth is that whenever you do cardio you will burn calories. The more effort you put in the quicker you will see results. To determine the best time to train you have to listen to your body. If you are not a morning person your body will find an early-morning session very hard. Doing it before lunch or after work will probably give you better results because you can put more effort in.

How to look good naked.

With our extensive range of weight loss products you can look fantastic with or without your clothes on!

The advanced formulas contain natural ingredients that help control your appetite and burn fat when you exercise; helping you to achieve the toned, sculpted body you've always dreamed of.

Say hello to the new you.

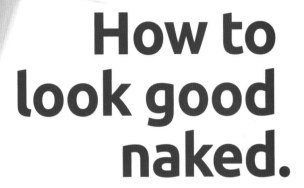

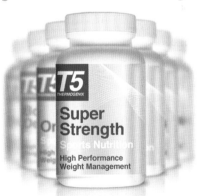

T5 THERMOGENIX

Super Strength

Sports Nutrition

High Performance Weight Management

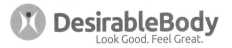

DesirableBody
Look Good. Feel Great.

www.desirablebody.co.uk
0845 459 6140

Get fired up
Metabolism boosters

Having a higher metabolism means that your body will burn more calories at rest. Here are the best ways to boost yours

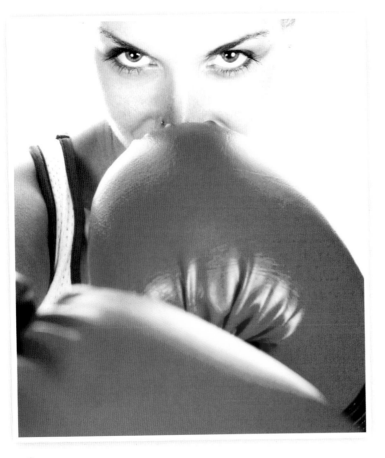

Most exercise will help raise your metabolism to some degree if done correctly, but some exercises are better than others for fat burning. It's the intensity of effort that causes the metabolism to speed up. High intensity may sound like a lot of hard work to produce good results, but interval training will give you a chance to switch between periods of working hard and recovering.

Many of us make the mistake of thinking that cardio alone is sufficient for weight-loss. While it will help us lose weight if we combine it with a healthy diet, our bodies will shrink but our shape will stay the same. In order to tone up and improve our bodyshape, we need to do some form of resistance training, which will boost our metabolism too.

Weight-training is the most effective exercise for boosting the metabolic rate. It makes you more metabolically active after a workout, due to blood flow and growth processes that occur in the muscles worked, whereas blood flow returns to normal relatively quickly after a cardio session. The more muscles you use to perform an exercise, the more your metabolism will be boosted.

Best exercises
The best exercises are those that work more than one muscle group. Basic exercises like bench presses, squats, lat pulldowns and leg presses are just a few multi-joint exercises that can create a greater degree of effort.

A basic weight-training routine to boost the metabolism would ideally comprise working all of your body's major muscle groups. Aim to perform three or four sets of ten to 12 repetitions per exercise. Ideally, you should train three times per week on non-consecutive days.

Other novel yet effective variations of weight-resistance exercise include

'Exercises that work more than one muscle group are the best metabolism-boosters'

one-legged exercises, such as a biceps curl or shoulder press. These are performed while standing on one leg, which increases muscle strength and endurance while also strengthening your core muscles.

You should consider, though, that the actual act of weight-training burns fewer calories in comparison with cardiovascular exercise. However, weight-training will lead to an increased muscle mass over time and maintaining lean muscle tissue will burn an increased amount of calories in the long term.

Fired up

Cardiovascular exercise is not only the best way to help reduce your bodyweight and fat percentage, it also plays a significant role in stoking your body's furnace. Anything that gets you moving and gets your heart pumping for a sustained period of time can be classed as cardio exercise. The key is to find something that has the fun factor and that will keep you motivated and stimulated. Cardio exercise helps boost your metabolism by teaching your body to burn fat while exercising and over time while resting as well.

There are a variety of activities for those bold individuals who want a challenging metabolism-boosting workout unlike anything else. For one, there are exercises that have you working out with skipping ropes. Jumping rope has a lot going for it as a metabolism stimulator.

Rope skipping is great for eating up the fat calories and assists in developing agility, coordination and balance, not to mention major improvements in cardio and muscular endurance.

Boot-camp workouts provide intense exercise sessions that challenge every muscle in your body and ignite your metabolism. By rapidly moving from exercise to exercise with little rest in between, you tone and firm muscles while getting a good cardio workout at the same time.

Combining martial arts with boxing gives you a fantastic cardio workout to create kickboxercise. You'll find yourself shadow boxing, skipping, using punch bags or teaming up with a partner to punch or kick focus pads. Both disciplines are considered two of the best high-intensity exercise classes to get you in great shape and skyrocket your metabolism, so kickboxercise will help you burn calories like no other cardiovascular workout.

With the popularity of the current crop of TV shows, dance classes are a great choice for people seeking a

Benefits of a faster metabolism

- Your body will be able to process the food you've taken in much faster and use up the calories, making sure that they won't linger in your body and eventually turn into fat.
- Once you're burning calories faster, you'll be able to eat more without feeling guilty. Still keep an eye on the quality, but you can be less concerned with quantity.
- With a faster metabolism, your body will perform more efficiently and you will have more energy.
- You'll burn more calories just by doing the activities you usually do; sitting in front of the TV will now burn 100!
- Your skin will be brighter and more radiant, and your face will be more alive with colour. With a faster metabolism, you will not only feel good but also look good.

31

'With a faster metabolism your body will be able to process the food you eat much faster and make sure it doesn't turn into fat'

powerful cardio workout but who also want to enjoy what they're doing. There is an abundance of non-traditional options, including classes where you'll 'shake your thing' to jazz, show tunes or funky pop. If you have a penchant for ethnic-style music and moves, there are all sorts of classes to select from too. Each dance form combines great bursts of endorphins and excitement, which leads to a positive increase in your body's thermostat.

Fusion fitness
This 'two for the price of one' form of exercise marries two or more activities into one session. Often, it's the merging of traditional and non-traditional exercises, and it's also a blend of cardio and toning and conditioning that will really help you maximise your outcome from each session.

Popular fusion exercises include Cy-Yo and Yogalates. Cy-Yo blends yoga and Spinning; it's ten minutes of yoga, 40 minutes of speed cycling on a stationary bike, then ten more minutes of yoga to cool down. Yogalates is a combination of yoga and Pilates and helps boost the metabolism by targeting the core muscles alongside muscle-elongating movements.

By following these tips and keeping your workouts as simple as possible you will be on your way to increasing your metabolism, building your muscle volume and losing weight. Even more importantly, you will become healthier and stronger too.

Avoid overtraining!

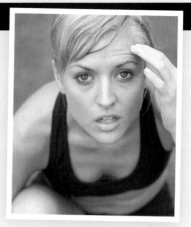

If you don't allow yourself sufficient recovery time from your cardio workouts, you may actually slow your fitness progress by limiting the effectiveness of each workout. This is commonly known as 'overtraining'.

A weaker immune system is one of the key indicators of overtraining and manifests itself in cold or flu-like symptoms, such as coughing, a runny nose or a sore throat.

Frequent cardio exercise can also increase the level of free radicals in the body. These are highly reactive atoms that can damage the body's cells. They can be formed when oxygen interacts with certain molecules, so there is a possibility of greater free-radical production with the greater oxygen uptake that is integral to cardio training. It may seem that cardio exercise increases damage to the body, but the body is able to adapt to regular activity by improving its defence system against damage.

A diet rich in vitamin E (found in nuts, seeds and fish oils), vitamin C (found in citrus fruits, green peppers and spinach) and beta-carotene (found in liver, egg yolk, milk, carrots and broccoli) will also help.

Blitz dimples
Beat cellulite

Regular cardio exercise will not only burn calories,
it will help attack stubborn fat and beat cellulite too

One of the main benefits of doing regular cardio exercise is that it can help beat cellulite. Like it or not, cellulite is just another word for fat, but as it is only fat, the good news is that we can improve its appearance by training and following a balanced diet.

Exercise will help you burn the existing fat in the fat cells that have caused your cellulite. It will also help you tone and firm the area that has been damaged by cellulite. It is important that you perform exercises that target the problem area to ensure that you are not wasting your time. Specifically, you want to be performing cardiovascular exercises, while performing small amounts of anaerobic activities to help tone the area.

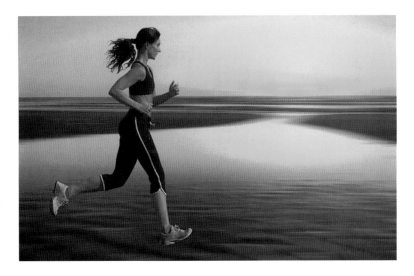

How can exercise beat cellulite?
- Do at least 30 minutes of cardio per day.
- Work up a sweat. If you are only glowing you are not working hard enough.
- Use a variety of cardio machines as they all work the muscles differently.
- Weight-bearing exercises, such as running and walking are better than non-weight-bearing exercises, such as swimming.
- Use interval training. The higher your level and the faster your speed the quicker you will get results.

Ten ways to minimise your cellulite
- Increase circulation to your cellulite areas by massaging the skin.
- A build-up of toxins in your body make it hard to break down fat, so try a detox diet for a month.
- Invest in a good anti-cellulite cream.
- Exercise at least three times a week. For every pound of extra muscles you have, you will burn an extra 50 calories a day.
- Avoid alcohol.
- Reduce drinks containing caffeine to a minimum.
- Reduce your salt intake.
- Reduce your sugar and sweet intake.
- Stop smoking. Tobacco smoke destroys vitamin C that is important to build collagen. Collagen is the building blocks of your skin. The weaker they become the more you will see your cellulite.
- Drink fennel tea or eat fennel. Fennel is a natural diuretic. The more water retention you have the more of your cellulite you will see.

You also need to tone your body with weights, or you could try a BodyPump class. It's important to make your weights routine regular, and ideally you need to be doing some form of resistance training three times a week for best results. Make sure you have a routine that works all of the muscles in the body.

33

Maximise your session

Good gym results

Make sure you get the best results from your gym workouts by using these guidelines, which will really boost your fitness routine

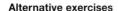

To get the most from your gym sessions, you need to be able to perform your exercise routine without any distractions. If you train at peak times and have to queue for machines it can be frustrating. So, instead of just standing around waiting, why not make the most of this time?

If you are waiting for the treadmill, for instance, you could train the same body parts by using the rower or the cross-trainer. If you are waiting for the upright cycle, which works the legs, you can also work the legs by using the recumbent cycle. If you are waiting for a particular piece of kit but someone is using it, you could always ask to 'work in' with them. This means that after they have performed their set, you do your set while they are having their rest and vice versa.

Alternative exercises
It's also good to be aware of alternative exercises you can do when you're not able to

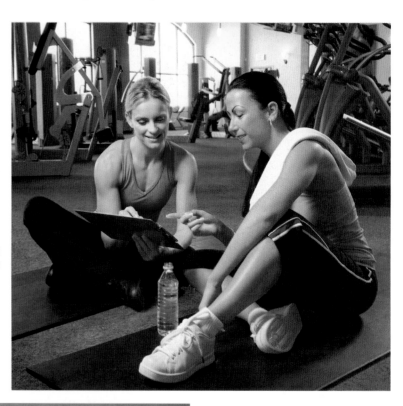

Machine	Body part trained	Alternative
Leg press	Front thighs	Leg extension
Seated hamstring curl	Rear thighs	Lying leg curl
Lat pulldown	Upper back	Seated row
Chest press	Chest	Pec deck
Cable pushdown	Rear upper arms	Bench dips
Preacher curl machine	Front upper arms	Dumbbell curls

use your usual machine, such as those shown in the table below.

You could also perform some of the same exercises on a stability ball. Lying on the stability ball on your back with your legs at 90 degrees and a pair of dumbbells in each hand will enable you to replicate the chest press exercise, for instance. You can also do squats

34

'The most effective cardio machines for weight-loss are the rower, treadmill and cross-trainer'

(for the front thighs) and lunges (for the rear thighs) without any exercise kit at all. There are plenty of alternatives, so if you find the gym crowded and aren't able to use the machines you need, speak to a gym instructor and ask them to recommend an alternative.

Cardio machines
The most effective cardio machines for weight-loss are the rower, treadmill and cross-trainer. Rowing is a brilliant way to burn lots of fat in a short space of time. Short bursts of high-intensity exercise are best here, so set yourself a distance to row, maybe 1,000 or 1,500 metres, and then see how fast you can complete the distance. Aim to beat your time whenever you visit the gym. Rowing can burn from 150 to 350 calories per 30 minutes.

For best results on the treadmill, aim to either run at a quicker pace for five to 15 minutes or jog at a steady speed for 20 to 30 minutes and you will burn fat fast. Running on the treadmill burns from 150 to 400 calories per 30 minutes, depending on your age, weight and present fitness level.

The cross-trainer works both the upper and the lower body, so will help you get your heart rate high and burn lots of calories, provided you push yourself and increase the resistance or pace (or both) for best results. The cross-trainer burns approximately 100 to 300 calories per 30 minutes.

The best gym classes for burning calories

Spinning – You're pedalling the whole time so you burn fat steadily, plus bursts of high activity get the heart, lungs and metabolism going. Calories burned per class: 350-700.

Circuit Training – There is very little rest as you're either working on a station or moving between stations, so the level of intensity remains high throughout the class. Calories burned per class: 300-500.

Boxing Fitness – This combines cardio exercise with punching bags and pads and offers a great fat-burning workout. You'll feel like you've really pushed yourself. Calories burned per class: 400-600.

35

Are you working hard enough?

To gauge your effort level, use the Rate of Perceived Exertion. On a scale of one to ten, work out how hard you are exercising by considering how easily you can breathe and if you are able to talk while working out. For weight-loss, work at a minimum of seven.

1 - Very light
2 - Fairly light
3 - Moderate
4 - Somewhat hard
5 - Hard
6
7 - Very hard
8
9
10 - Very, very hard

Rev up your fitness
Running plans

Running can burn up to 15 calories per minute, depending on your age, weight and fitness level, so get started and watch the pounds melt away

If you're new to running you need to build up your time slowly. Here's a selection of workouts to suit everyone's schedule.

Getting started

■ Warm up by walking gently and then increasing your walking to a speed that requires a bit of effort – a good swing of the arms and a longer stride length will get your heart going and warm you up thoroughly. Make sure you warm up for 3-4 minutes.

■ Once you've mastered each programme you can make them tougher by slowly increasing the intensity of each stage. If you're running on a treadmill, increase the speed for each part of your workout. If you're running outdoors you'll need to judge how to push yourself a little harder for each part of the workout.

■ To get the best results with these workouts you need to make sure that by the end of any periods of faster running you're really ready to take a breather and slow down. If you could carry on at that speed, you're not pushing it hard enough for these tougher sections.

■ Always cool down following your running. You can do this by gradually decreasing the intensity of your exercise from a run to a fast walk to a slow walk. A cooldown is key for recovery from running.

36

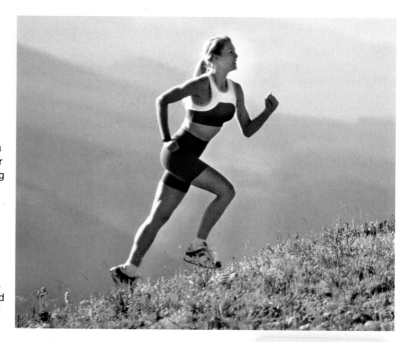

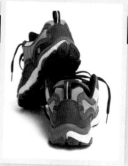

Good running technique

■ Run in an upright position. Keep your head up and your eyes ahead of you.
■ Use your arms as well as your legs.
■ Keep your stomach tight and your shoulders relaxed at all times.
■ Breathe deeply as you run.
■ Aim for good posture.

How often? If you follow these plans and run two or three times a week you'll soon see results. You can run up to five days a week but have at least two days off a week and rest after a challenging workout.

15-minute plan for beginners

CALORIE BURN 180

- 2 minutes faster running
- 2 minutes moderate-speed running
- 2 minutes faster running
- 2 minutes moderate-speed running
- 2 minutes faster running
- 2 minutes moderate-speed running
- 2 minutes faster running
- 1 minute slow running to recover

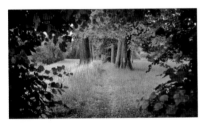

Making your 30-minute plan more advanced

With this plan your objective is to reduce the time spent running at a moderate speed for each 5-minute round and increase the time spent running at a faster speed. Once you've successfully completed a split of 4 minutes and 1 minute a few times, alter the split to 3.5 minutes moderate: 1.5 minutes fast. Then move onto 3 minutes moderate: 2 minutes fast and so on until you can manage 1 minute moderate: 4 minutes faster running for each 5-minute section.

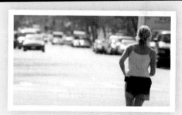

20-minute plan for beginners

CALORIE BURN 240

- 2 minutes slow running
- 1 minute moderate-speed running
- 1 minute faster running
- 1 minute running as fast as you can
- 1 minute fast running
- 1 minute moderate-speed running
- 5 minutes slow running
- 1 minute moderate-speed running
- 1 minute faster running
- 1 minute running as fast as you can
- 1 minute fast running
- 1 minute moderate-speed running
- 3 minutes slow running

20-minute plan for intermediates

CALORIE BURN 275

When you are confident running for 20 minutes consistently, the next challenge is to make sure you use your training time effectively. This simple routine will guarantee that you're always challenging your fitness levels and making progress.
- 10 minutes moderate-speed running
- 5 minutes running at a slightly quicker speed, judging your pace so that you can just about maintain this pace for the full 5 minutes
- 5 minutes moderate-speed running

30-minute plan for intermediates

CALORIE BURN 350

- 4 minutes moderate-speed running
- 1 minute fast running
- Repeat x 6

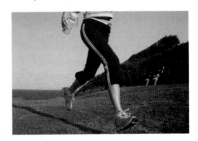

Enjoy the ride

Cycling plans

Cycling is an ideal fat-burner, and the best part is you can cycle anywhere – in the gym, outside, on the way to work, or at a leisurely pace at the weekend

If you're new to cycling you'll be looking for a varied training plan so you don't get bored. If you're cycling outdoors your mind should be stimulated as you observe what's going on around you. If you're training on a stationary bike in the gym, focus on these workouts closely and the time will fly by.

If you are using the stationary bike in the gym, make sure you have a good upright posture and you also need to ensure that the seat height is right for you. The seat should be level with your hips when you are standing sideways on and your knee should not be locked out when you extend your legs.

Getting started

■ Warm up for each plan by pedalling gently for 3-4 minutes. Sit upright on the bike and keep your shoulders back and relaxed as you ride.

■ To increase the intensity of any workout, increase the levels on the stationary bike or begin pushing a bit harder on the tough sections earlier in the routine; for example, at the start of a faster section rather than saving your effort for the end. You'll know you're working hard if your legs are burning, so aim to get to this stage quicker as you get more confident with each plan.

■ Cool down by slowing your pedal rate very gradually over the course of 3-4 minutes.

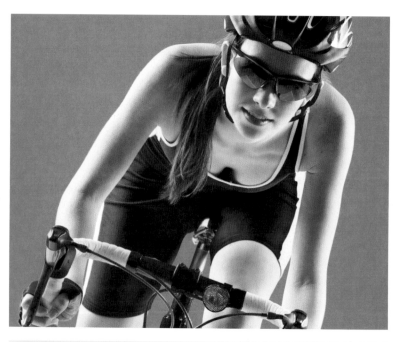

Good cycling technique

■ Make sure the seat height is level with your hips.

■ Maintain good posture.

■ Don't lock your knees out on extension.

■ Keep your hips still; if they are rocking from side to side, then your seat height is too high.

■ Pull your tummy in to activate your core.

■ Wear a heart-rate monitor, as this will help you measure your progress.

How often? For maximum weight-loss aim for three to four workouts per week using a combination of the different plans. Aim to do each plan in turn rather than focusing only on the shorter plans.

15-minute plan for beginners

Indoors
- 3 minutes moderate cycling – level 4
- 2 minutes faster cycling – level 5
- 3 minutes moderate cycling – level 4
- 2 minutes faster cycling – level 5
- 3 minutes moderate cycling – level 4
- 2 minutes faster cycling – level 5

Outdoors
15-minute route that includes hills. Pedal hard up the hills and coast down the hills to recover.

20-minute plan for beginners

Indoors
- 3 minutes easy cycling – level 3
- 3 minutes moderate cycling – level 4
- 2 minutes faster cycling – level 5
- 1 minute tough cycling – level 6
- 1 minute hard cycling – level 7
- 3 minutes easy cycling – level 3
- 3 minutes moderate cycling – level 4
- 2 minutes faster cycling – level 5
- 1 minute tough cycling – level 6
- 1 minute hard cycling – level 7

Outdoors
20 minutes along a route that includes some hills. Push your legs hard up and down the hills – there's no coasting in this plan!

20-minute plan for intermediates

Indoors
- 3 minutes moderate cycling – level 4
- 3 minutes faster cycling – level 5
- 3 minutes tough cycling – level 6
- 3 minutes hard cycling – level 7
- 3 minutes tough cycling – level 6
- 3 minutes faster cycling – level 5
- 2 minutes moderate cycling – level 4

Outdoors
Cycle for a period of 10 minutes, gradually increasing your pace. Then gradually decrease your pace for the second 10 minutes. If you gauge the pace correctly for the first half, you should still feel that you're working hard all through the second half of the workout despite the fact the intensity or pace is reducing.

30-minute plan for intermediates

Indoors
- 3 minutes moderate cycling – level 4
- 3 minutes tough cycling – level 6
- 3 minutes faster cycling – level 5
- 3 minutes hard cycling – level 7
- 3 minutes tough cycling – level 6
- 1 minute full-effort cycling – level 8
- 3 minutes tough cycling – level 6
- 3 minutes hard cycling – level 7
- 3 minutes faster cycling – level 5
- 5 minutes moderate cycling – level 4

Outdoors
This is a stepped programme so cycle for 30 minutes along a route where you can access a variety of hills with as much variation in the incline as possible. Aim to keep your rhythm consistent for each different hill.

Making your 30-minute plan more advanced

You can make this plan more advanced in three ways:
1. Increase the speed of your cycling (revs per minute) for each part of the plan.
2. Increase the level for the minute of full-effort cycling halfway through the plan.
3. Increase the level at which you begin the plan, as this will raise the intensity of each phase.

39

Hit the pool
Swimming plans

Swimming is ideal if you're injured, or you don't like going to the gym –
it burns fat fast without jarring the body and offers great results

 Want to lose weight with swimming? Follow these plans to get results.

Getting started

■ Warm up with some gentle lengths of the pool for around 5 minutes. Use this time to relax your shoulders and concentrate on breathing deeply as well as regularly.

■ If you need to increase the intensity of each programme because it has become too easy, you can increase the speed of your fast swimming or decrease the duration of the slower-speed recovery swimming, e.g. 3 lengths of steady-speed recovery swimming instead of 4.

■ Cool down from each workout with a couple of very gentle lengths.

Essential kit

■ Swimsuit
■ Goggles
■ Swimming cap
■ Towel

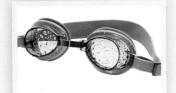

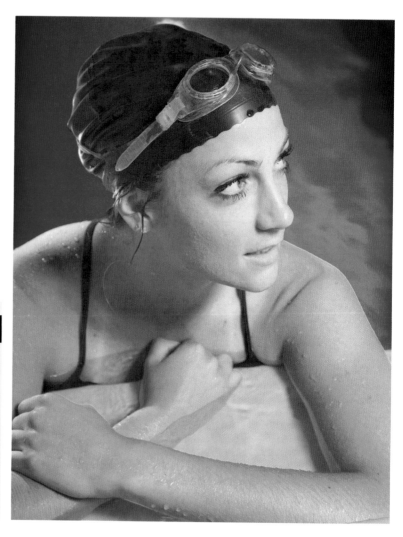

40

How often? For maximum weight-loss, aim to swim at least three times a week with at least one rest day between swims.

15-minute plan for beginners

CALORIE BURN 105

- Swim 4 lengths at a steady pace
- Swim 2 lengths at a fast pace
- Repeat for the rest of the workout

20-minute plan for beginners

CALORIE BURN 140

- 5 minutes steady-pace swimming
- 5 minutes fast-pace swimming
- 5 minutes steady-pace swimming
- 5 minutes fast-pace swimming

20-minute plan for intermediates

CALORIE BURN 200

- Swim 4 lengths at a steady pace
- Swim 1 length at a fast pace
- Swim 4 lengths at a steady pace
- Swim 2 lengths at a fast pace
- Swim 4 lengths at a steady pace
- Swim 2 lengths at a fast pace
- Swim 2 lengths at a steady pace
- Swim 2 lengths at a fast pace
- Swim 4 lengths at a steady pace
- Swim 1 length at a fast pace
- Swim 4 lengths at a steady pace

30-minute plan for intermediates

CALORIE BURN 250

- Swim 10 lengths at a steady pace
- Swim 4 lengths at a fast pace
- Swim 4 lengths at a steady pace
- Swim 4 lengths at a fast pace
- Swim 10 lengths at a steady pace
- Swim 2 lengths at a fast pace
- Swim 2 lengths at a steady pace
- Swim 2 lengths at a fast pace
- Swim 10 lengths at a steady pace

41

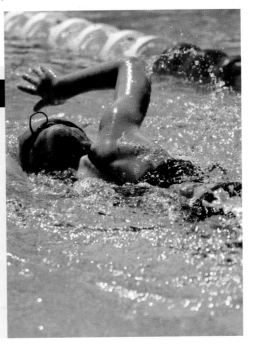

Making your 30-minute plan more advanced

- Every time you do your 30-minute workout, aim to reduce the number of lengths you swim for the major recovery sections by a length at a time from 10 lengths to 4 lengths.
- Aim to progressively increase the speed of your fast-paced swimming.
- Aim to progressively increase the speed of your steady-paced swimming.

- Over time, you can increase the number of lengths that you swim at a fast pace for the first 'sprint' section of the plan. Ultimately you should aim to increase this part to swim 10 lengths at a faster pace before you start your period of recovery.

Magic machine

Cross-trainer plans

The cross-trainer works the entire body without the impact of the treadmill, and it burns plenty of calories, too

 For optimum results on the cross-trainer make sure you practise good technique:

■ Stand upright on the machine with your stomach tight and keep your shoulders relaxed.

■ Work your arms and legs evenly and share the load between pushing and pulling with either side of your body.

■ Keep your hips and shoulders forwards throughout your programme and avoid rolling your shoulders from side to side or swaying too much at the hips.

■ Regularly tightening your bottom muscles will help keep you in position.

Getting started

■ Warm up on the cross-trainer with 3-4 minutes of steady movement. Check your posture during this time and make sure that you get into a steady rhythm.

■ If you want to make any of these programmes a little tougher, simply increase the levels for each part of the workouts when you're ready or increase the intensity of each section of the workout by speeding up your movement. Just be careful that if you speed up the movement, you don't compromise the technique.

■ Cool down on the cross-trainer with 3-4 minutes of steady movement and take deep breaths to help speed up your recovery.

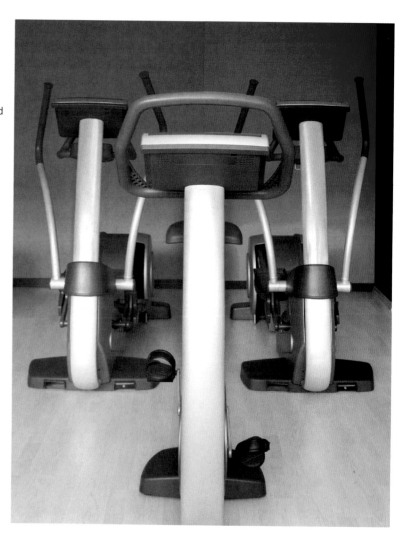

How often? For best weight loss results you'll need to get on the cross-trainer three or four times a week. Make sure that you have at least two rest days each week – if you push yourself hard enough with your training, you'll need them.

15-minute plan for beginners

CALORIE BURN 75

- 3 minutes at a comfortable level
- 3 minutes at a comfortable level +1
- 3 minutes at a comfortable level +2
- 3 minutes at a comfortable level +1
- 3 minutes at a comfortable level

20-minute plan for beginners

CALORIE BURN 100

- 5 minutes at a comfortable level
- 4 minutes at a comfortable level +1
- 3 minutes at a comfortable level +2
- 2 minutes at a comfortable level +3
- 1 minute at a comfortable level +4
- 5 minutes at a comfortable level

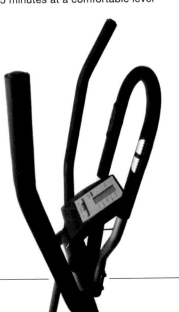

20-minute plan for intermediates

CALORIE BURN 150

- 3 minutes at a comfortable level
- 3 minutes at a comfortable level +2
- 3 minutes at a comfortable level +3
- 3 minutes at a comfortable level +4
- 3 minutes at a comfortable level +3
- 3 minutes at a comfortable level +2
- 2 minutes at a comfortable level

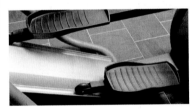

30-minute plan for intermediates

CALORIE BURN 200

- 2 minutes at a comfortable level
- 2 minutes at a comfortable level +1
- 2 minutes at a comfortable level +2
- 2 minutes at a comfortable level +3
- 2 minutes at a comfortable level
- 2 minutes at a comfortable level +1
- 2 minutes at a comfortable level +2
- 2 minutes at a comfortable level +3
- 2 minutes at a comfortable level +4
- 2 minutes at a comfortable level
- 2 minutes at a comfortable level +1
- 2 minutes at a comfortable level +2
- 2 minutes at a comfortable level +3
- 2 minutes at a comfortable level +4
- 2 minutes at a comfortable level +5

Making your 30-minute plan more advanced

- Increase the speed on each part of the plan.
- Begin the plan at a higher level and work through it on increased levels for each section.
- Stick with the same comfortable level but increase the intensity of the tougher sections. So, instead of comfortable +1 to 3, aim for comfortable +2 to 4 and so on.

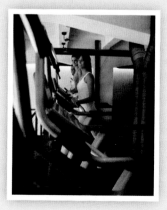

43

Full-body blaster

Rowing plans

Rowing is a cardio exercise that works both the upper and lower body and burns serious calories. It's also a great muscle toner

When you start rowing, it's important to pay good attention to your technique. Follow the guidelines in the box opposite, or the guidelines on the machine itself, and you can't go wrong. If you're still unsure, ask a member of staff at your gym to point you in the right direction. Once you've cracked the technique you can be sure of a really good workout. You should also find out how to use the console on the rowing machine so that you can set up some of the specific workouts described here.

Getting started

■ Warm up on the rowing machine with 2 minutes of steady rowing, and then 1 minute of rowing with a strong pull on the handles while you straighten your legs, followed by a slow forward movement to recover between each stroke. This will ensure that you're thoroughly warm before you start.

■ To make each programme harder increase your pace for the faster periods of rowing and the slower periods of rowing. Practise more powerful strokes instead of increasing your stroke rate dramatically.

■ Cool down with 2 minutes of gentle rowing at the end of each programme. Practise an upright posture at this stage so your lungs are fully open and you recover quicker.

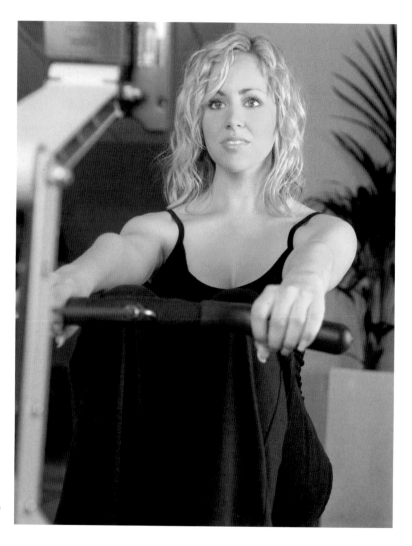

How often? Try rowing three times a week for maximum weight-loss. If you push yourself on every visit you'll be amazed at the results you'll see.

15-minute plan for beginners

CALORIE BURN 150

- Row at a steady pace for 4 minutes
- Set the rower for a 250m sprint
- When you're ready, row the 250m as fast as you can and note your time
- Recover for 2 minutes
- Repeat the 250m sprint and note down your time
- Recover for 2 minutes
- Repeat the 250m sprint and note down your time
- Row at a steady pace for 4 minutes

15-minute plan for intermediates

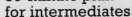

CALORIE BURN 250

- Row at a steady pace for 4 minutes
- Set the rower for a 250m sprint
- When you're ready, row the 250m as fast as you can and note your time
- Recover for 2 minutes
- Repeat the 250m sprint and note down your time
- Recover for 2 minutes
- Repeat the 250m sprint and note down your time
- Row at a steady pace for 4 minutes

20-minute plan for beginners

CALORIE BURN 200

- Row at a steady pace for 4 minutes
- Row at a fast pace for 4 minutes
- Row at a steady pace for 3 minutes
- Row at a fast pace for 3 minutes
- Row at a steady pace for 2 minutes
- Row at a fast pace for 2 minutes
- Row at a steady pace for 1 minute
- Row at a fast pace for 1 minute

30-minute plan for intermediates

CALORIE BURN 375

- Row at a steady pace for 4 minutes
- Row at a faster pace for 1 minute
- Row at a steady pace for 4 minutes
- Row at a faster pace for 2 minutes
- Row at a steady pace for 4 minutes
- Row at a faster pace for 3 minutes
- Row at a steady pace for 4 minutes
- Row at a faster pace for 4 minutes
- Row at a steady pace for 4 minutes

Making your 30-minute plan more advanced

Over time, replace time spent rowing at a steady pace for time spent rowing at a faster pace. Your aim is to end up with a 30-minute plan where you row for sections of four minutes at a faster pace with only one minute at a steady-pace recovery before you speed up again.

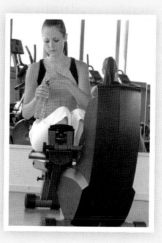

Safe rowing technique

- Sit with your legs bent, arms straight, heels slightly lifted and eyes forward.
- Straighten your legs and bend your arms as you pull back.

- Keep your legs straight but not locked out at the knees.
- Straighten your arms and begin to bend your legs, returning to the start position.

45

Jump to it
Skipping plans

Serious about ditching those extra calories? Then take up skipping, it's a huge fat-burner and very effective with the right technique

If you're new to skipping, choose a rope that is either plastic or leather – these turn better and are easier to use than the old-fashioned nylon ropes.

Getting started
■ Warm up with short bursts of skipping. Begin with a round of 20 and then increase to 30 and then 40.
■ If you need to make these workouts tougher you can do so by changing your technique. Begin skipping with a small hop between each jump of the rope. This is a good, slow rhythm to start with. When you're confident with this you can start to lose the hop between jumps and practise one jump for every turn of the rope without the 'recovery' hop between jumps. Once you've perfected this you can try alternate leg skipping, which is the kind of skipping that boxers use and requires a quick rhythm with the rope and good coordination.
■ Cool down with slow skips, reducing the number in each round from 40 to 30 to 20 to 10.

Essential kit

■ Skipping rope
■ Trainers
■ Bottle of water

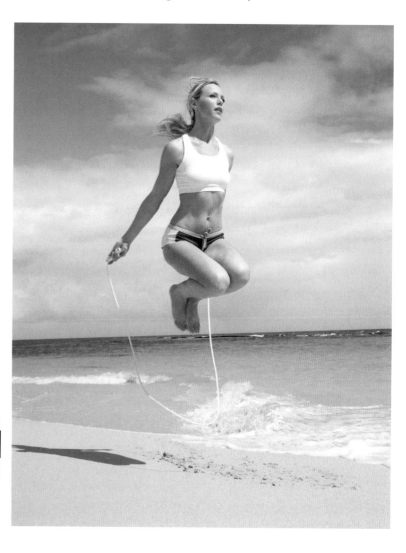

How often? If you really want great results with weight-loss, try skipping five days a week and have the other two days off.

5-minute plan for beginners

CALORIE BURN 50

- Skip for 30 seconds
- Rest for 30 seconds
- Skip for 60 seconds
- Rest for 30 seconds
- Skip for 1.5 minutes
- Rest for 30 seconds
- Skip for 30 seconds

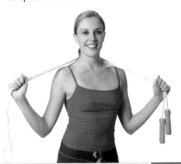

15-minute plan for intermediates

CALORIE BURN 200

- Skip for 30 seconds
- Rest for 30 seconds
- Complete 50 skips
- Rest for 30 seconds
- Complete 75 skips
- Rest for 30 seconds
- Complete 100 skips
- Rest for 30 seconds
- Continue increasing the number of skips you do in each round by 25 until you have been skipping for a total of 15 minutes

20-minute plan for intermediates

CALORIE BURN 250

- Skip for 60 seconds
- Rest for 60 seconds
- Skip for 1.5 minutes
- Rest for 60 seconds
- Skip for 2 minutes
- Rest for 60 seconds
- Skip for 2.5 minutes
- Rest for 60 seconds
- Skip for 3 minutes
- Rest for 60 seconds
- Skip for 4 minutes
- Rest for 60 seconds

47

10-minute plan for beginners

CALORIE BURN 100

- Skip for 30 seconds
- Rest for 30 seconds
- Skip for 30 seconds
- Rest for 30 seconds
- Skip for 30 seconds
- Rest for 30 seconds
- Skip for 30 seconds
- Rest for 30 seconds
- Skip for 30 seconds
- Rest for 30 seconds
- Skip for 60 seconds
- Rest for 60 seconds
- Skip for 60 seconds
- Rest for 60 seconds
- Skip for 60 seconds

Good skipping technique

Good technique when skipping will mean that you can get a better rhythm and your workouts will be much more enjoyable without lots of stopping and starting.
- Stay upright at all times with your tummy pulled in, keeping your shoulders back and down.
- Be light on your feet as much as you can by using your knees and your ankles to keep your rhythm.
- Breathe in deeply while you skip.

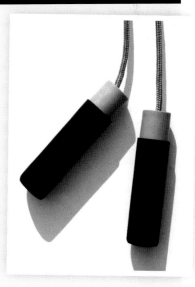

Square up
Cardio combat

Shadow boxing is a fun, fat-burning workout that really gets results

If you get bored on the treadmill, the cross-trainer or the rower and normal aerobics classes just don't do it for you, then you can perform your own combat workout at home. Combat burns many calories, as it involves short, sharp bursts of movement and it's also a great toner for the upper body. If you want to do combat moves at home, you can do so without any exercise kit whatsoever. Forget boxing gloves, pads or a punch bag, shadow boxing is highly effective if you do it right and perform the moves regularly enough to get results. Try these moves three to four times per week and you'll soon be burning calories. Put on some loud music for added motivation and you'll love it!

- For your warm-up go through all the moves slowly.
- Do ten repetitions on each side for each exercise.
- Repeat the sequence but increase your speed.
- Complete three to five times.
- As a cooldown complete each move slowly.

48

Squat to uppercut
Thighs, bottom, stomach and shoulders

- Stand with good posture, your feet slightly wider than hip-width apart.
- Keep your elbows tucked in, your fists covering your chin and your knees soft.
- Bend your knees and squat back, push through your legs and bring your elbow across your body and up.
- Pull your elbow back, squat down and repeat on the other side.
- As you push back to the standing position, try and rotate from your waist as you punch up.

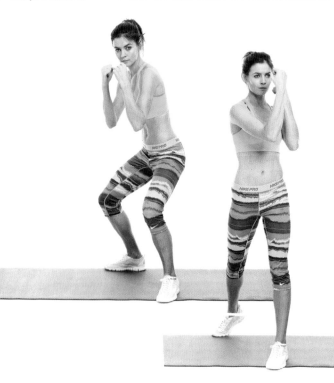

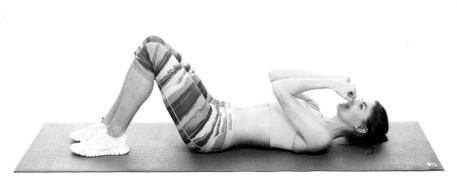

Ab, jab and cross

<u>Stomach, chest and shoulders</u>

■ Lie on the floor on your back with your knees bent and feet flat.
■ Position your hands in front of your chest with your elbows tucked into your sides.
■ Slowly curl up, exhaling as you do so, bringing your shoulders off the floor.
■ Pause at the top and punch your right fist out over your left knee and then your left fist over your right knee.
■ Slowly return to the start position and repeat, leading the punches with the opposite fist.

49

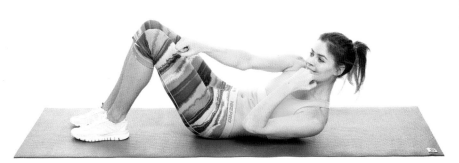

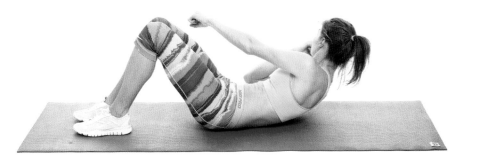

Grab and high knee

Stomach, hips and bottom

■ Standing with good posture, take a small step back with your right foot.
■ Reach up with both your hands.
■ As you pull your hands down bring your right knee up to meet your arms.
■ Return to the start position.
■ Repeat on the opposite leg.

50

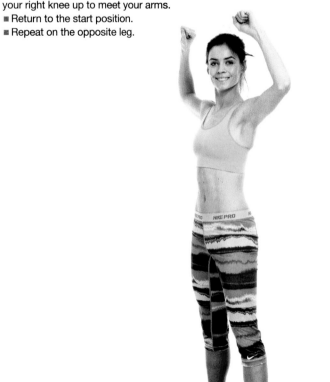

Jab, cross and hook

Stomach, chest and shoulders

■ Standing with good posture, rotate to the side (if you're
right-handed rotate clockwise, if left-handed, anticlockwise),
tuck your chin in, keep your elbows tight to your body
and bring your fists up to your chin and shoulders.
■ Punch straight out with your left hand (jab), quickly pull
back and punch straight out (cross) with your right hand.
■ Pause, bring up your right elbow and rotate your body from your
waist, punching around and across with your left arm (hook).
■ Reset your position, jab, cross and hook with the other
side. Alternate the hooks on each combination.

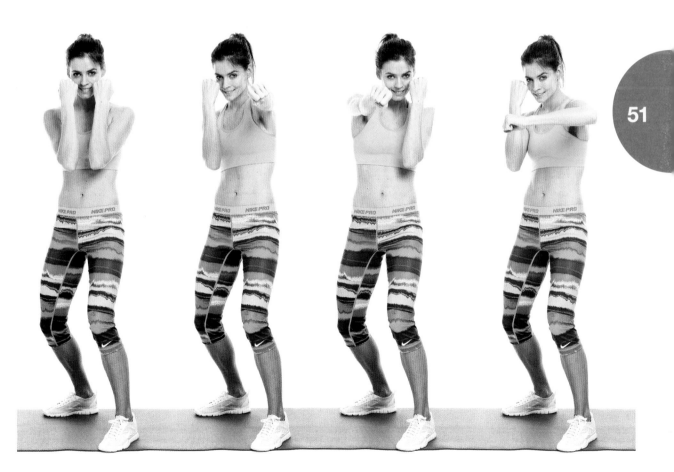

51

Side kick

<u>Thighs and stomach</u>

- Start with your feet hip-width apart.
- Lean over to the left, tuck your chin in, keep your elbows tight to your body and bring your fists up to your chin and shoulders.
- Lift your right foot off the floor, then lift your knee up towards your elbow.
- Keeping your balance on your left leg, kick out to the side with the right foot.
- Pull your leg back in and place it back on the floor.
- Step back to the start position.
- Repeat on the other side keeping the number of repetitions equal.

52

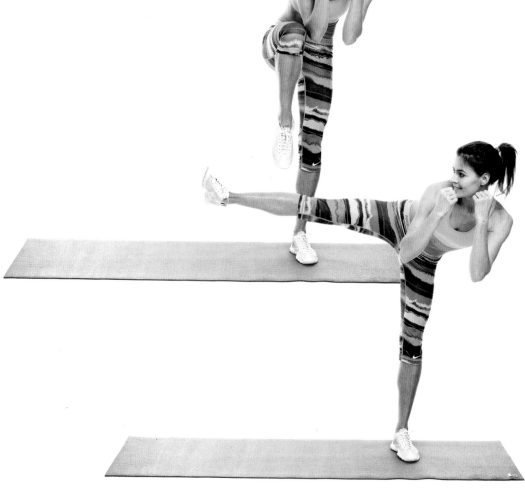

Rotating side lunge

Thighs, bottom and lower back

■ With good posture, plant your feet roughly one-and-a-half times shoulder-width apart and squat down.
■ Extend your right leg straight out to the side, keeping your left knee bent. Sink your hips back, keeping your shoulders back and your chest lifted.
■ Bend your left arm and bring it up to shoulder height, extending your right arm out to the side.
■ Push back through your left leg and repeat on the opposite side.

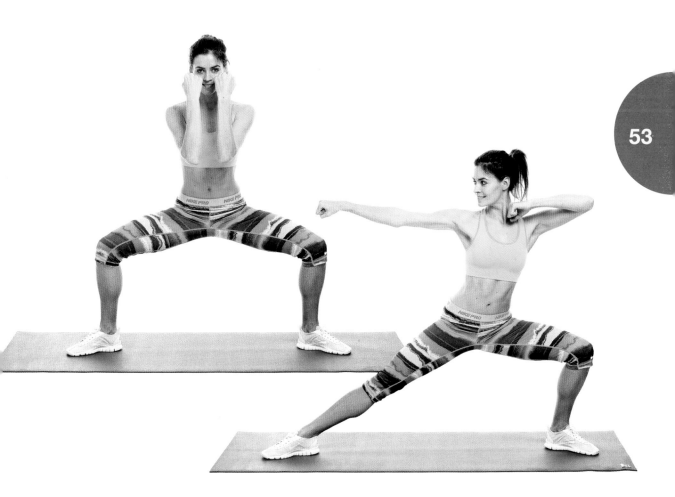

53

How to follow these workouts...

On the pages that follow there are workouts for every body part, but you don't have to do every single exercise!

It is best to do a full-body workout rather than a split routine if you are a beginner or an intermediate exerciser, as if you skip a routine you won't miss out on training certain body parts.

Beginners: If you are a beginner, choose one exercise per body part from each section and repeat it for six weeks before choosing a different exercise for each body part.

Intermediates: If you already work out, choose two exercises per muscle group and split the workout into two programmes and repeat them for six weeks before choosing two different exercises per body part.

Advanced: If you are super-fit, design three different programmes (three exercises from each section) and follow these split routines over three separate training days:

- Chest, bottom and stomach
- Legs, back and waist
- Arms and core

Add a posture exercise (or two or three depending on your fitness level) to a fourth day of training if you have time. Alternatively, you can add it to the arms and core routine.

Duration: For great results, work out for an hour in total. Each toning routine will take approximately 20-30 minutes, so you will have plenty of time for a cardio routine and stretching at the end.

54

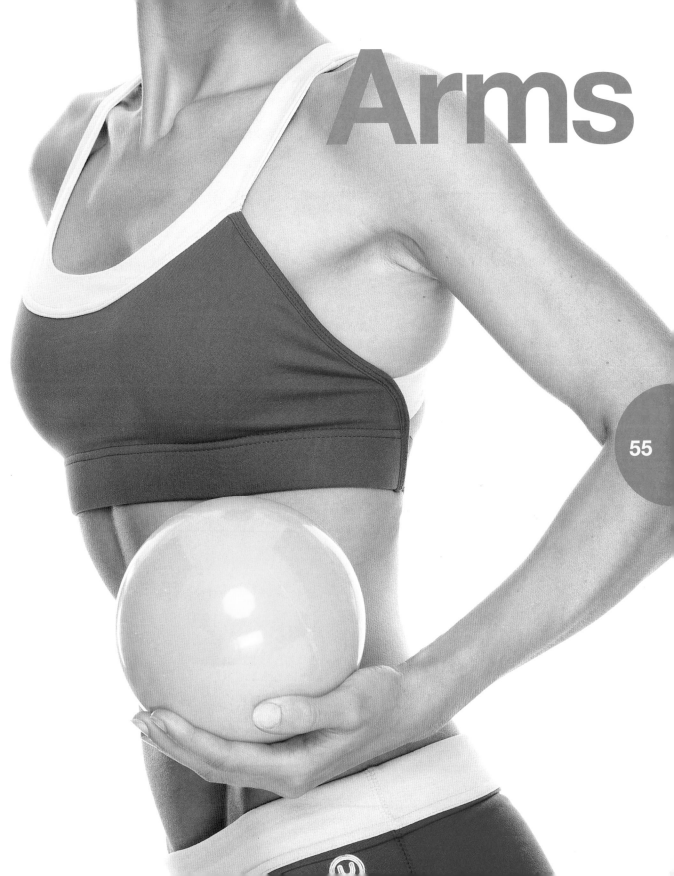

Arms

55

Biceps curl

Front of upper arms

- Hold a weight in each hand with your palms facing forward.
- Bend your arms, lifting the weight towards your armpits.
- Keep your elbows tucked into your sides.

56

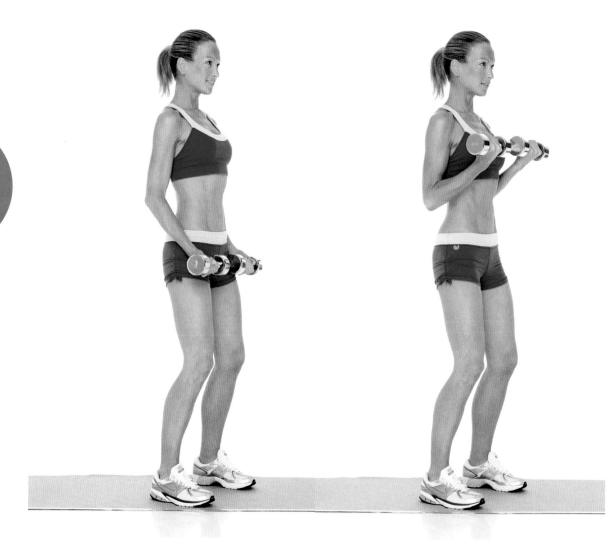

Press-ups with one arm forward

Front of upper arms, chest and shoulders

■ Kneel on the floor, keeping your left hand just behind the line of your shoulder and your right hand in front.
■ Ensure that your body is parallel with the floor.
■ Bend your elbows, lowering your chest to the floor.
■ Lower down to where you feel comfortable.
■ Push back up.
■ Repeat on the other side with your left hand in front.

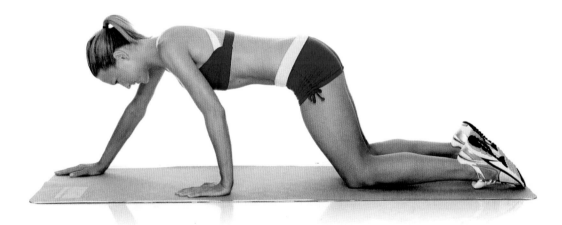

57

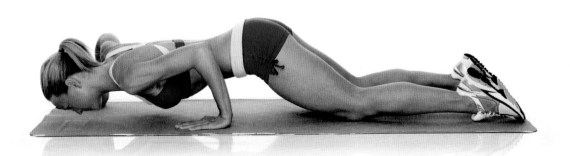

Shoulder press

<u>Shoulders</u>

- Stand up straight with good posture.
- Hold a weight in each hand next to your shoulders with your palms facing forwards.
- Extend your arms up to the ceiling but don't lock your elbows.
- Lower your arms back to the starting position.

58

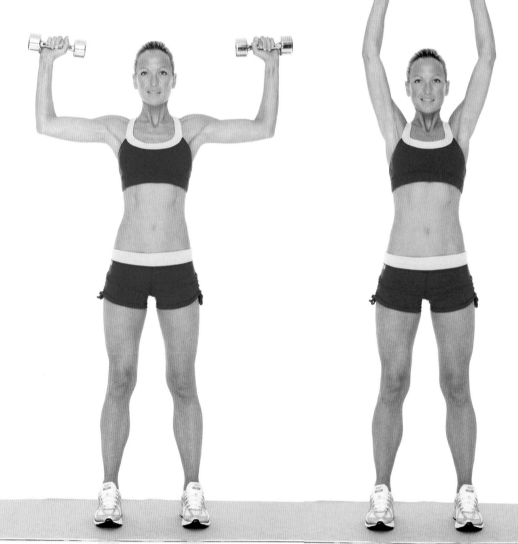

Front raises

<u>Shoulders</u>

■ Stand with your feet hip-width apart, holding a weight in each hand with your palms facing down.
■ Keep your arms in front of your thighs with a slight bend in your elbows.

■ Lift your left arm up to shoulder height.
■ Lower with control.
■ Ensure that you don't swing your body to lift the weight up.
■ Alternate with the other arm.

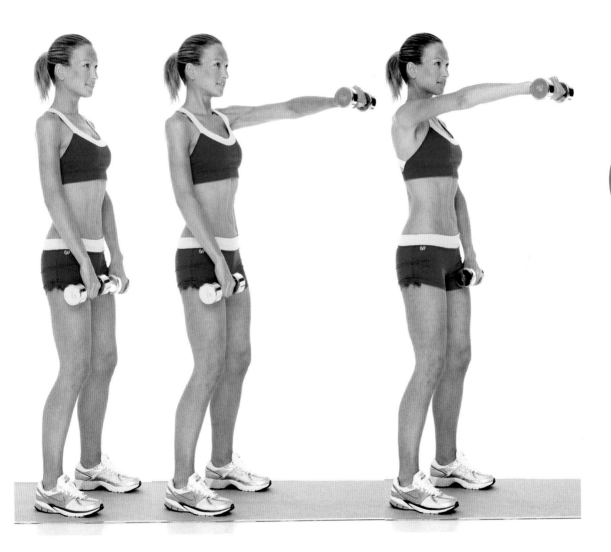

59

Kneeling overhead triceps extension

Back of upper arms

- Kneel on the floor with your back upright.
- Hold a weight in one hand and extend it up to the ceiling.
- Lower the weight to your shoulder blade.
- Extend your arm up to the ceiling but don't lock your elbow.
- Repeat on the other side.

Tip: Support your elbow with your opposite hand, if needed.

60

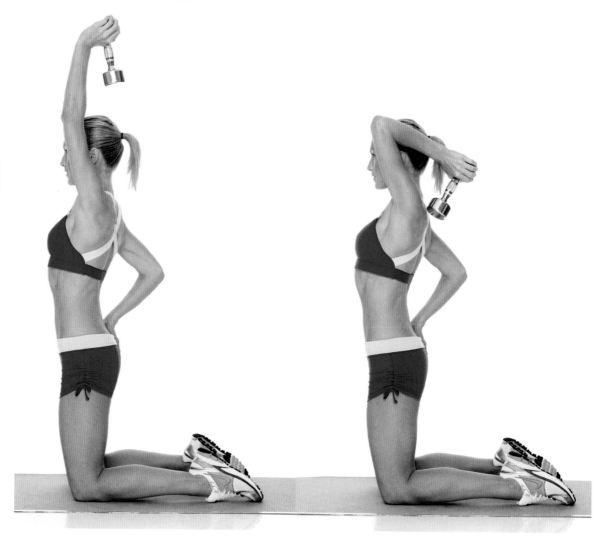

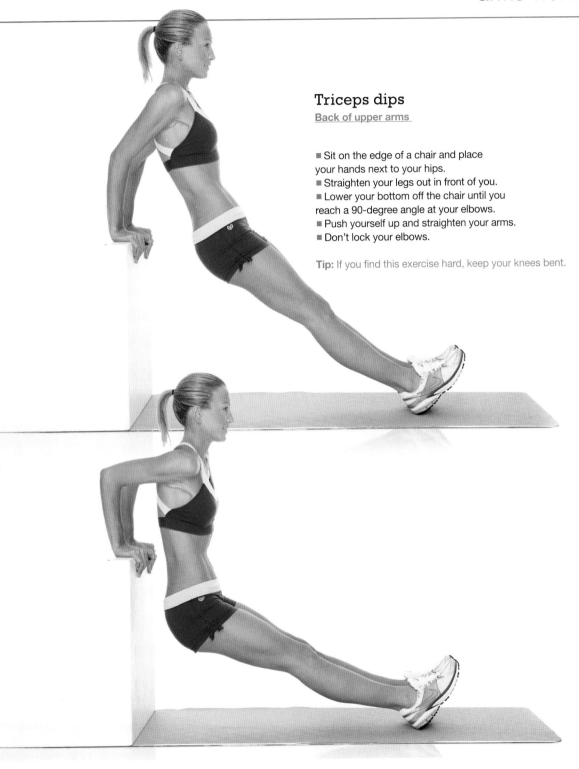

Triceps dips
Back of upper arms

- Sit on the edge of a chair and place your hands next to your hips.
- Straighten your legs out in front of you.
- Lower your bottom off the chair until you reach a 90-degree angle at your elbows.
- Push yourself up and straighten your arms.
- Don't lock your elbows.

Tip: If you find this exercise hard, keep your knees bent.

61

Arms guidelines

REPS AND SETS:

Beginners: 2 sets of 10 to 15 repetitions using a light weight
Intermediate: 2 to 3 sets of 20 repetitions using a light weight
Advanced: 3 sets of 10 to 15 repetitions using a moderate weight

62

About the arms

Muscles work in pairs – when one muscle contracts, the opposite muscle relaxes, so it's important to work opposite muscle groups in equal balance. This means that when you work your biceps (front upper arms), you need to ensure that you work your triceps (rear upper arms) too. Don't skip one and do the other. Exercising your arms will not only make them look shapely and toned in T-shirts and sleeveless tops, but it will also make daily tasks like lifting heavy shopping much easier.

For best results

■ Perform the exercises slowly. Don't speed up as this will cause you to use momentum rather than strength.
■ When doing biceps curls, keep your upper body still. Don't swing your back – if you can't lift the weight without doing this then lower the weight.
■ Never sacrifice quality for quantity.

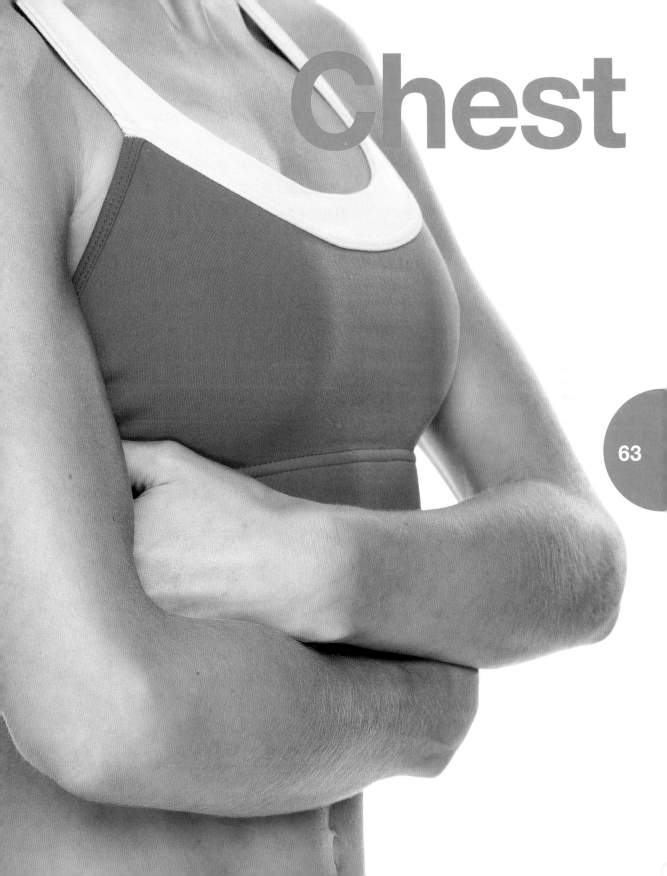

Chest

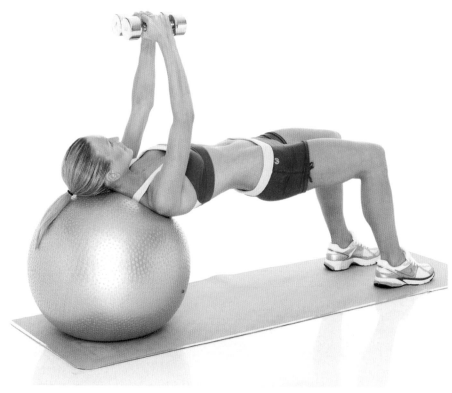

Stability ball dumbbell fly

Chest and armpits

- Lie on a stability ball with your head and shoulders supported and your knees at right angles.
- Holding a weight in each hand, extend your arms up to the ceiling with your palms facing each other. This is the start position.
- Keep a slight bend in your elbows.
- Open your arms until the weights are in line with your shoulders.
- Return to the start position.

Tips:
- Keep your tummy and bottom tight.
- Keep a straight back.

64

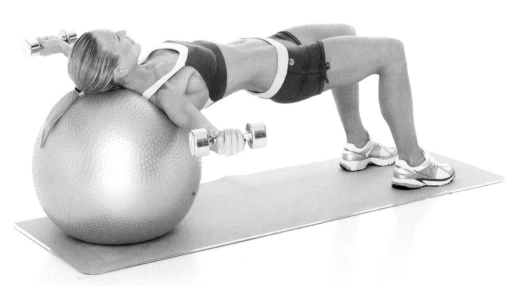

Stability ball pullover

Stomach, chest, back and arms

- Lie with your back on a stability ball and your knees at right angles.
- Holding a weight in each hand, extend your arms up to the ceiling with your palms facing away from you. This is the start position.
- Lower your arms above your head while keeping them straight.
- Return to the start position.

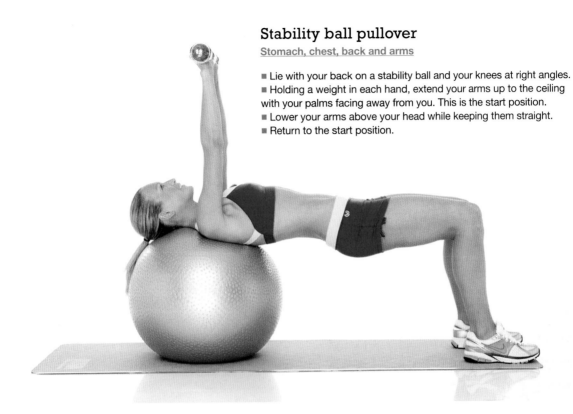

65

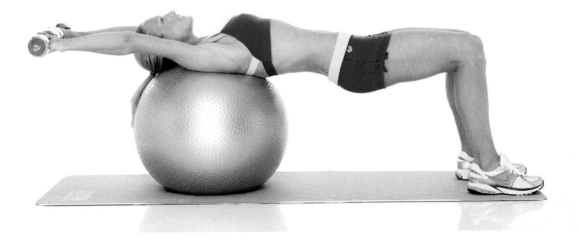

Stability ball press-up with hands on ball

Chest, arms and core stability

- Lie with your chest on a stability ball.
- Place your hands next to your chest on the ball, keeping your fingers spread open.
- Straighten your arms and lift your body off the ball.
- Lower with control.

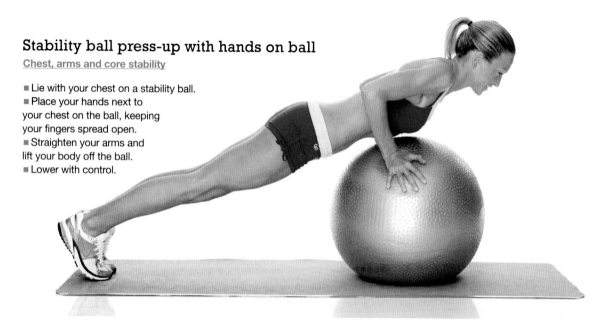

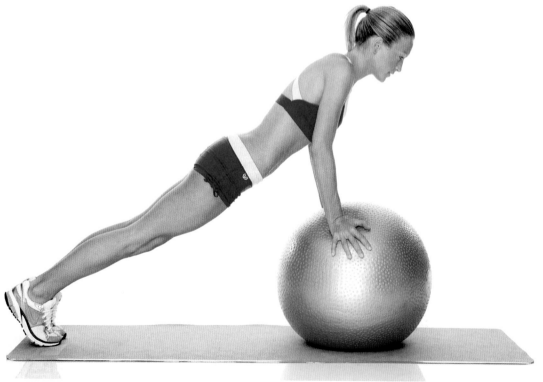

Dumbbell chest press

Chest and arms

- Lie on your back with your knees bent, holding a weight in each hand.
- Bring the weights up to shoulder height, with your palms facing away from you.
- Extend your arms up to the ceiling.
- Lower the weights until your elbows touch the floor.
- Extend your arms back up to the start position.

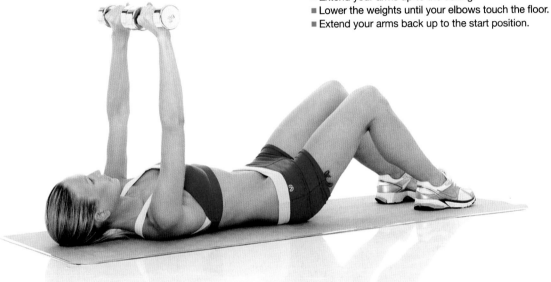

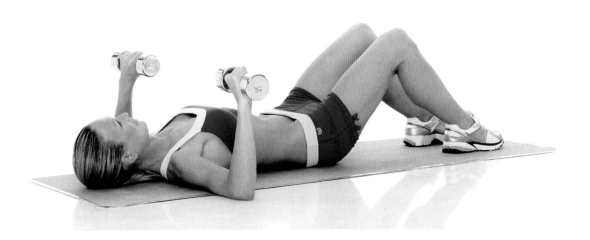

67

Box press-ups

<u>Chest and arms</u>

- Kneel on all fours.
- Place your hands slightly further apart than your shoulders.
- Bend your elbows and lower your chest to the floor.
- Extend your arms back up, without locking the elbows.

Tip: Keep your back straight and your tummy tight.

68

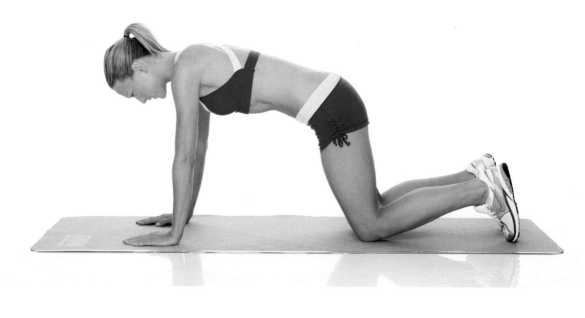

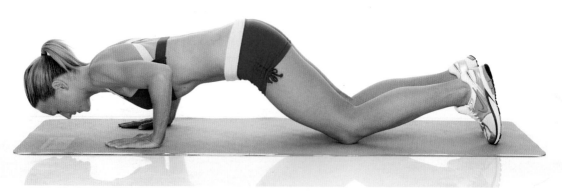

Incline fly against a stability ball

<u>Chest and arms</u>

■ Place a stability ball firmly against a
wall and lean back against it.
■ Hold a weight in each hand with
your palms facing inwards.
■ Extend your arms up until the weights
meet in the middle, but don't lock your
elbows. This is the start position.
■ Open your arms sideways until the
weights are level with your shoulders.
■ Return to the start position.

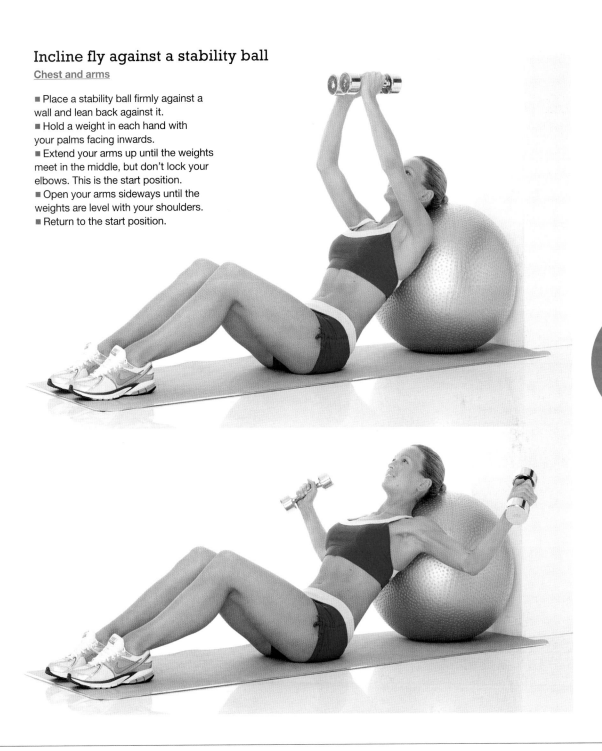

69

Chest guidelines

REPS AND SETS:
Beginners: 2 sets of 10 to 15 repetitions using a light weight
Intermediate: 2 to 3 sets of 20 repetitions using a light weight
Advanced: 3 sets of 10 to 15 repetitions using a moderate weight

About the chest
Working your chest will make the whole area feel much firmer. Your shoulders and triceps (rear upper arms) will also get a workout when you work your chest, allowing you to burn even more calories. Don't forget to wear a sports bra whenever you exercise. The ligaments in the chest are not elastic and once you stretch them they will be permanently stretched, leading to a saggy bust.

For best results
- Do the exercises slowly and don't use momentum.
- If you are using dumbbells, never hold them above your face. They should be level with the midline of the chest.
- Gym machines that work the chest include the pec deck, chest press and bench press.

70

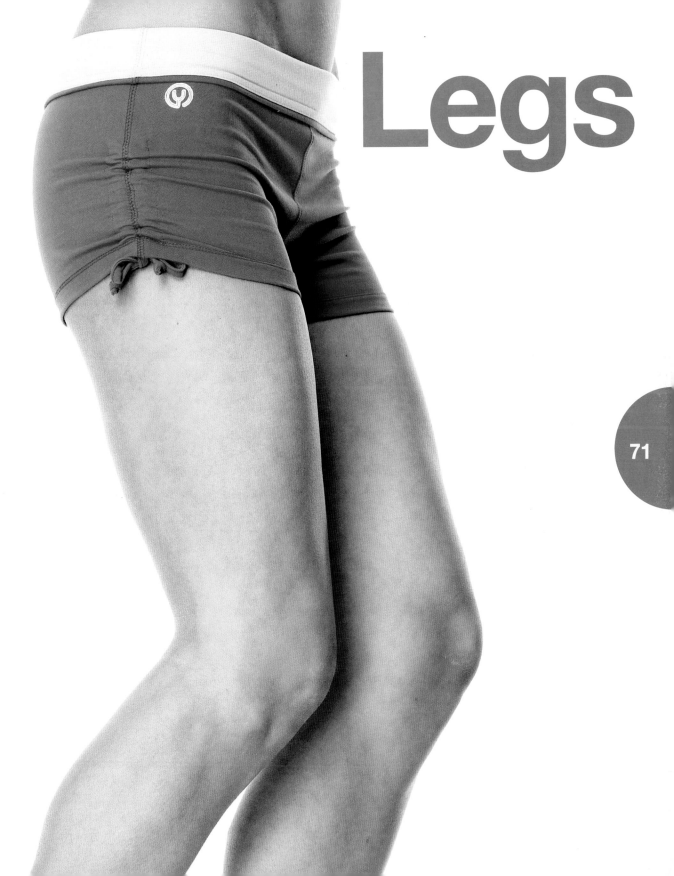

Legs

71

Outer thigh side leg lift

Outer thighs

- Lie on your side in a straight line with your legs on top of each other.
- Lift your top leg up towards the ceiling.
- Lower your leg with control.
- Pull your belly button into your spine and squeeze your bottom throughout the movement.
- Repeat on the other side.

72

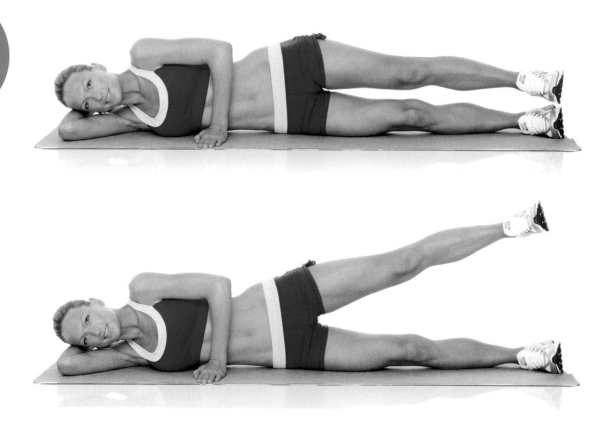

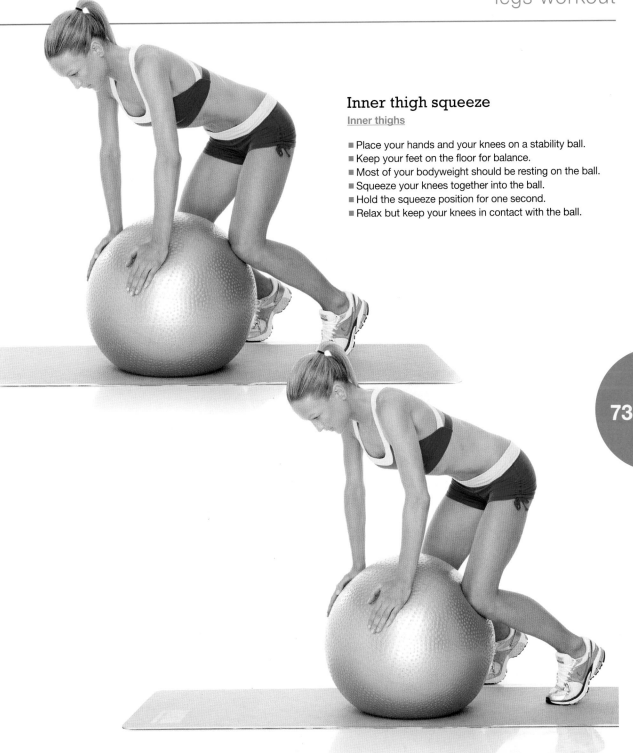

Inner thigh squeeze

Inner thighs

- Place your hands and your knees on a stability ball.
- Keep your feet on the floor for balance.
- Most of your bodyweight should be resting on the ball.
- Squeeze your knees together into the ball.
- Hold the squeeze position for one second.
- Relax but keep your knees in contact with the ball.

73

Plié

Hips, thighs, calves, bottom and stomach

■ Stand with your feet slightly wider than shoulder-width apart, toes pointing out at 45 degrees. Put both hands on your hips.
■ Bend your knees to 45 degrees and lift your heels off the floor, while squeezing your bottom tight.
■ Slowly lower your heels back and straighten your legs.

Tip: Hold onto a chair for balance, if necessary.

74

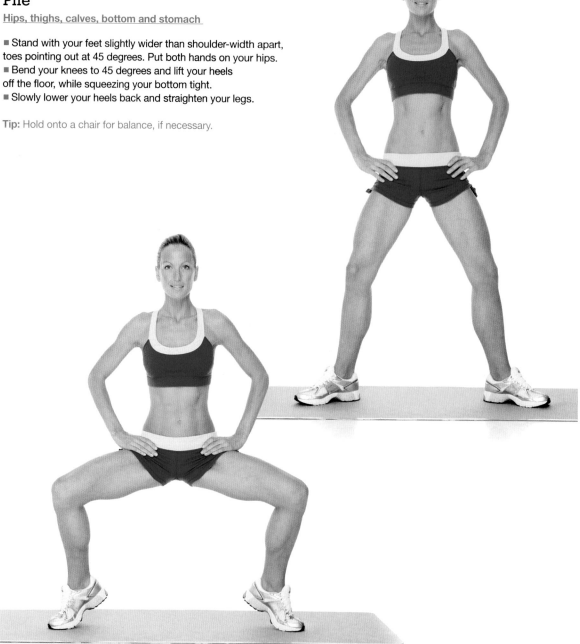

Dumbbell leg curl

<u>Rear thighs</u>

■ Lie down on your stomach, fold your arms
and rest your forehead on your arms.
■ Hold a weight between your feet so that the top
end of the weight rests on the soles of your shoes.
■ Squeeze your feet together and curl your legs
up towards your bottom.
■ Slowly lower with control but don't rest on the floor.

75

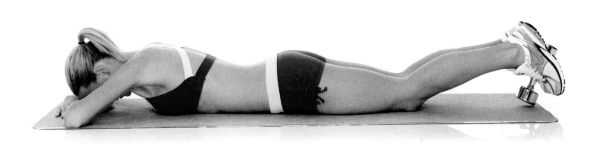

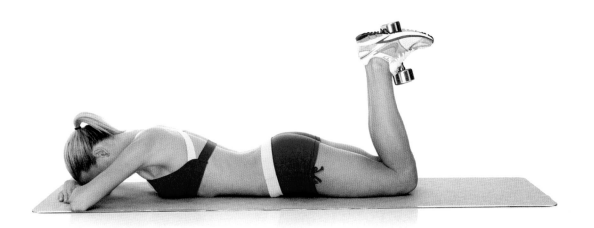

Calf raise with dumbbells

<u>Calves and ankles</u>

- Stand with your feet hip-width apart with a dumbbell in each hand.
- Raise yourself onto your tiptoes, keeping your weight evenly distributed between your big toe and little toe on each foot.
- Keep your shoulders relaxed and knees slightly bent throughout this exercise.
- Lower your heels back to the ground slowly.

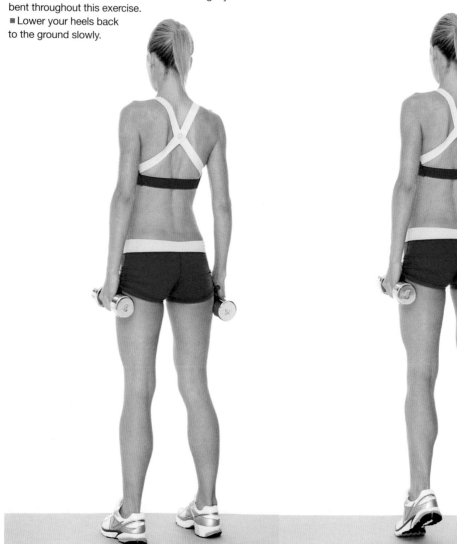

76

Lunge with punching

Legs, arms and shoulders

■ Stand with your feet together while
holding a light weight in each hand.
■ Keep your elbows bent at 90 degrees
with your palms facing each other.
■ Lunge forwards with your right foot and simultaneously
punch your left arm forwards, followed by your right arm.
■ Step backwards and repeat with your left foot.

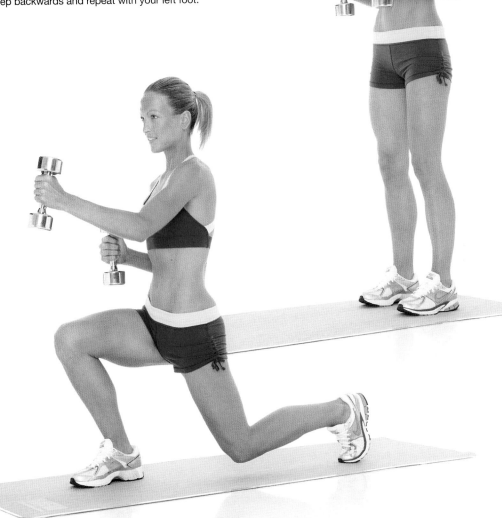

77

Legs guidelines

REPS AND SETS:

Beginners: 2 sets of 15 repetitions using a light weight
Intermediate: 2 sets of 20 repetitions using a light weight
Advanced: 3 sets of 20 repetitions using a moderate weight

About the legs

Toned and shapely legs not only look great on a night out, but having strong legs will also help you with your cardiovascular exercise. Whether you prefer running, cycling or classes, strong legs are the foundation of a fit, lean body and will help you keep going during a particularly challenging run or cycle.

For best results

■ Perform the exercises slowly. Don't speed up as this will cause you to use momentum rather than strength.
■ Gym machines that work the legs include the leg press, leg extension and seated hamstring curl.
■ Gym classes that will work the legs include cardio combat and circuit training, where you will be doing lots of squats and lunges.

78

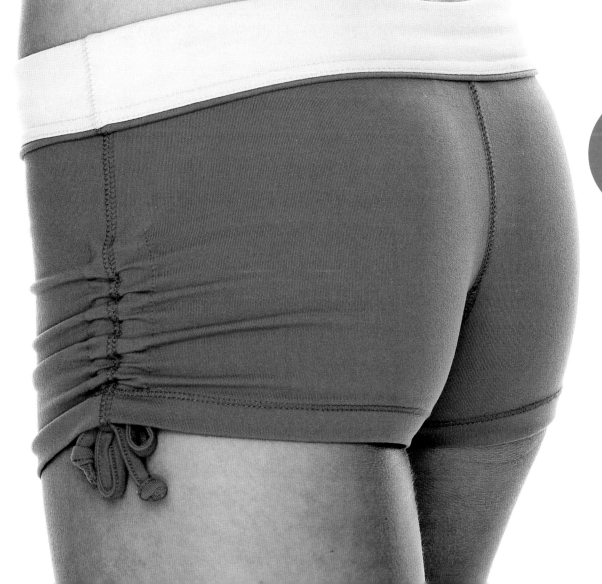

Bottom

Basic bridge

<u>Bottom and thighs</u>

■ Lie on your back with your knees bent, your feet shoulder-width apart and your arms by your sides.
■ Contract your stomach muscles and squeeze your bottom while lifting it off the floor.
■ Lift until you form a straight line between your knees, hips and shoulders.
■ Hold the top position for three seconds before lowering back to the starting position.
■ Don't rest on the floor in between repetitions.

80

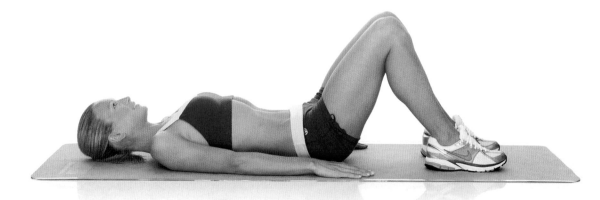

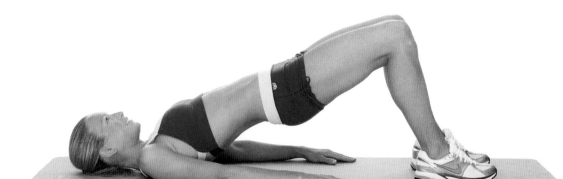

Kneeling side-kick

Bottom

- Kneel on all fours and extend your left leg sideways, tilting your head and body to the left.
- Lift your left leg off the floor to hip level.
- Bend and straighten your knee to perform a kicking move.
- Complete one set and repeat on the right leg.

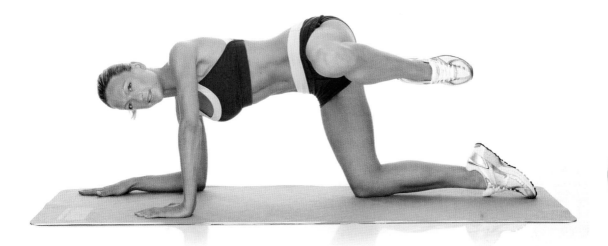

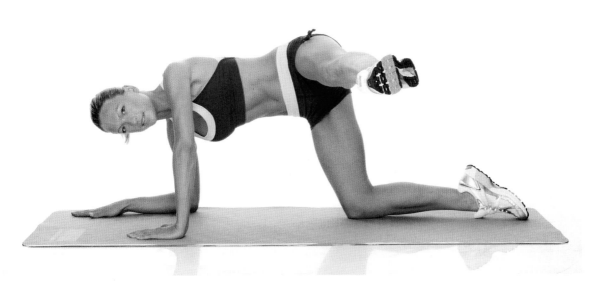

81

Step-ups

Thighs and bottom

- Stand at the bottom of the stairs.
- Place your right foot on the second step.
- Push up through your thighs and lift
your left leg onto the second step.
- Reverse the movement and
return to the start position.
- Repeat the movement on the opposite leg.

Tip: Stay tall throughout the movement.

82

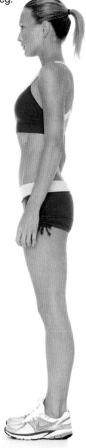
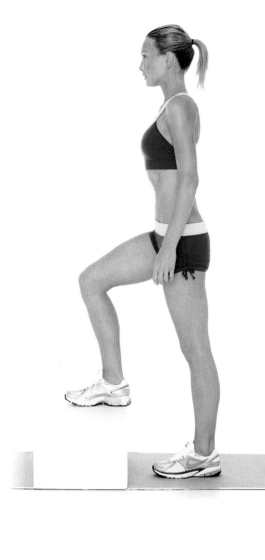

Single-leg squat

<u>Thighs, bottom and lower back</u>

- Stand up straight with your feet hip-width apart, toes pointing forwards.
- Lift one foot off the floor and soften the supporting knee.
- Push the hips back, bend the knee and keep the chest up.
- Pause at the lowest point and push back up to the start position.
- Repeat on the other leg.

Tips:
- Try to position yourself in front of a mirror. When you lift your foot off the floor check to make sure your hips and shoulders are still level.
- Keep the hip, knee and ankle stacked above one another.

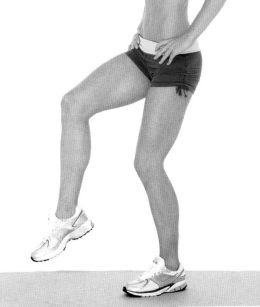

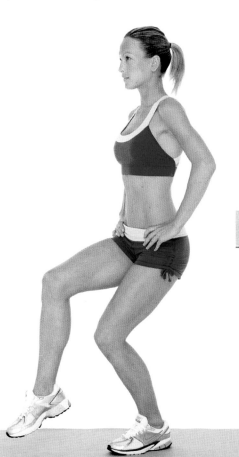

83

Single-glute bridge on stability ball

Bottom, lower back and rear thighs

- Lie on the floor with a stability ball in front of you.
- Place your hands by your sides with your palms turned down, keeping your shoulders relaxed.
- Bend your knees and place your feet on the stability ball.
- Lift your left foot so that your leg is straight and your knees are together.
- Keeping your hips level and your right foot on the ball, raise your bottom off the floor. Slowly lower it towards the floor, pause and push your hips back up into the air.
- Swap legs and repeat.

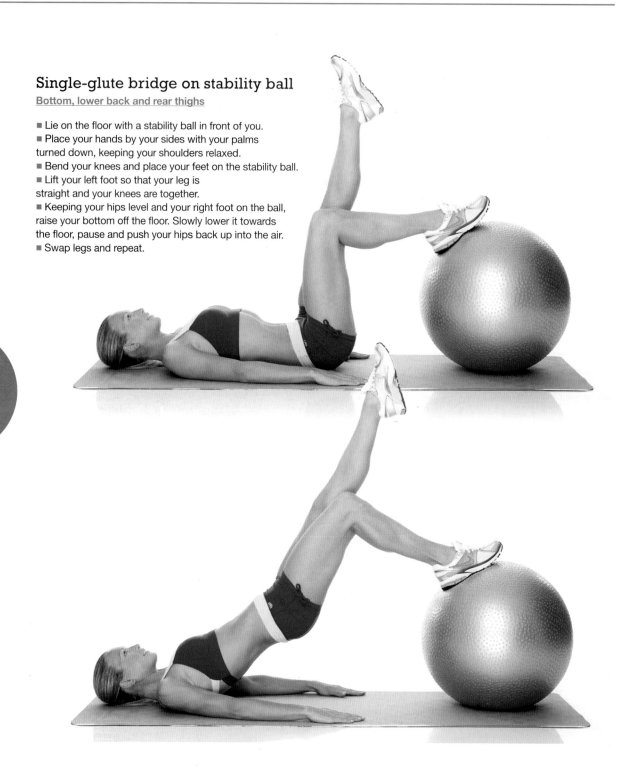

84

Glute lifts on a stability ball

Bottom

- Lie with your stomach on a stability ball.
- Bend your left knee.
- Keep your right foot and your

hands on the floor for balance.
- Push your left heel up towards the ceiling.
- Hold the top position for a few seconds.
- Lower until your knee touches the ball.
- Repeat one set on your left leg

before repeating on the right.

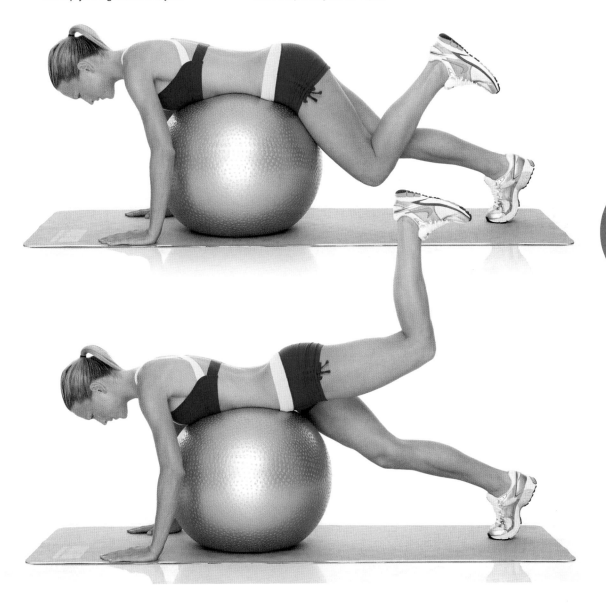

85

Bottom guidelines

REPS AND SETS:
Beginners: 2 sets of 15 repetitions
Intermediate: 2 sets of 20 repetitions
Advanced: 3 sets of 20 repetitions

About the bottom
You can shape and tone your bottom by doing our exercises, but you can also firm up the glutes by using the cross-trainer machine in the gym or by walking on an incline on the treadmill. Walking uphill fires the glutes and encourages them to work effectively.
Having strong glutes protects your body from injury, as weak glutes means that other muscles have to work harder to do their job. Weak glutes have often been associated with knee injuries, for instance.

For best results
■ Do the exercises slowly and don't use momentum.
■ MBT shoes, FitFlops and Reebok's EasyTone shoes all fire the glutes and hamstrings when you walk.

86

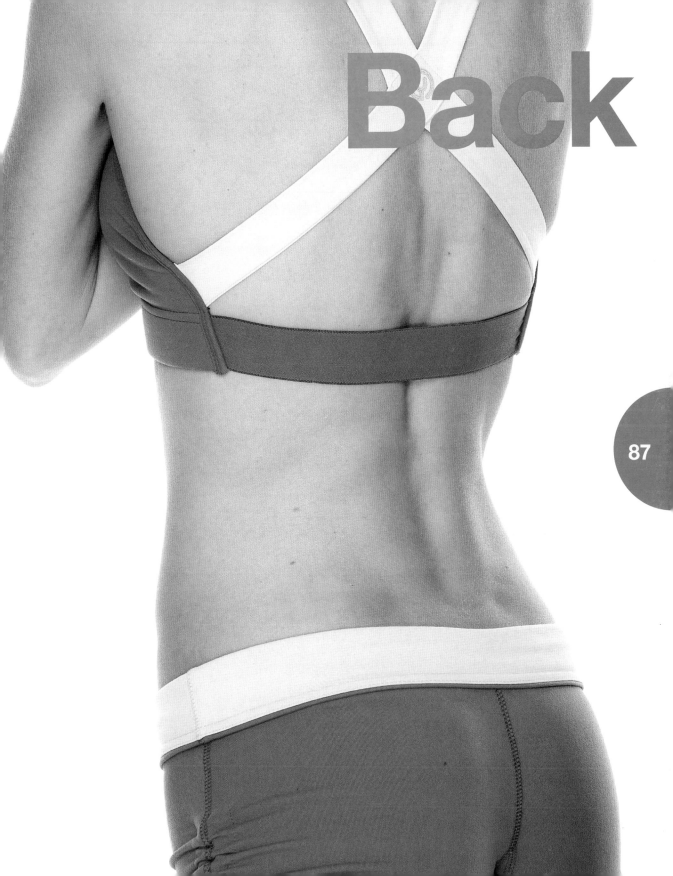

Back

Prone back extension

Back

- Lie on your stomach with your arms by your sides.
- Keep your palms facing up.
- Lift your upper body and arms off the floor.
- Rotate your palms down and
squeeze your shoulder blades.
- Hold the position for a few seconds
before lowering your body.
- Keep your feet on the floor at all times.

88

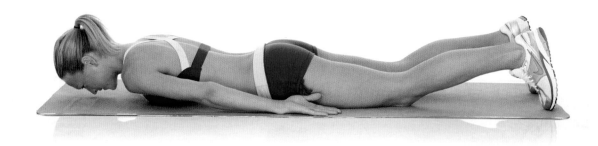

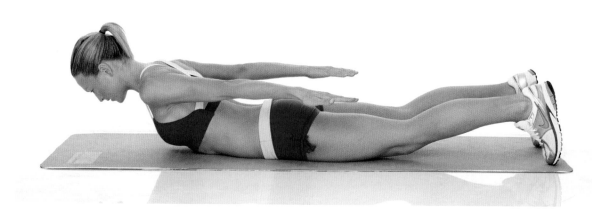

Stability ball cobra

Back and bottom

■ Lie with your stomach on a stability ball and position your arms in a 'Y' shape, palms facing the floor. This is the start position.
■ Keep looking at the floor to avoid lifting your chin too high and putting pressure on your neck.
■ Squeezing your bottom, slowly lift your chest off the ball. Draw your arms back, squeezing your shoulder blades and turning your thumbs up to point towards the ceiling.
■ Hold this position for a count of three to five seconds and slowly release, returning to the start position.

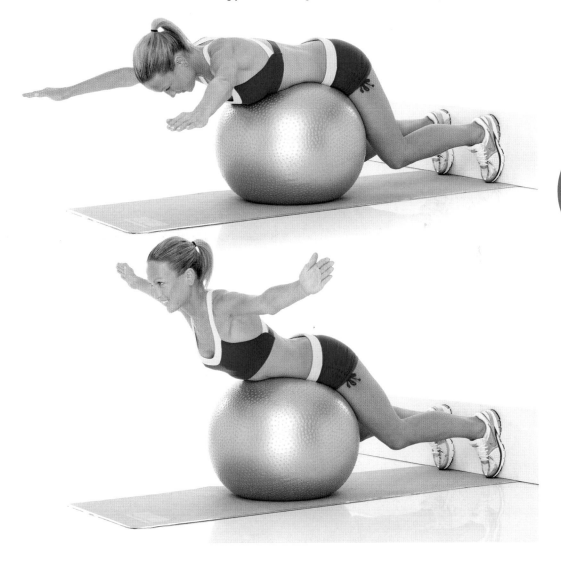

89

90

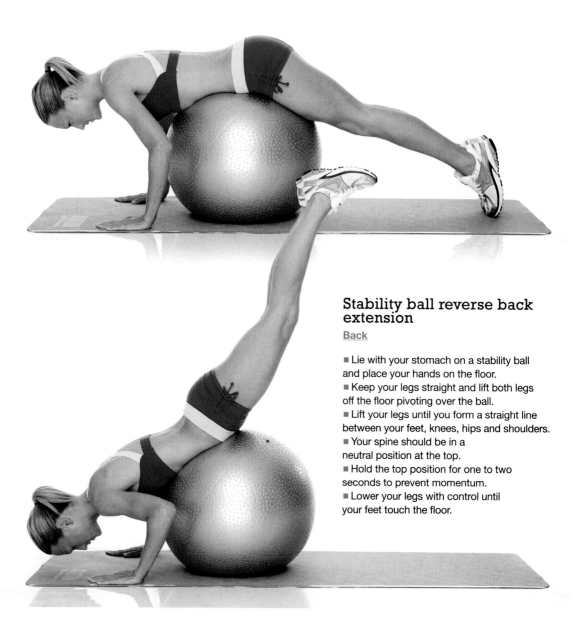

Stability ball reverse back extension

Back

■ Lie with your stomach on a stability ball and place your hands on the floor.
■ Keep your legs straight and lift both legs off the floor pivoting over the ball.
■ Lift your legs until you form a straight line between your feet, knees, hips and shoulders.
■ Your spine should be in a neutral position at the top.
■ Hold the top position for one to two seconds to prevent momentum.
■ Lower your legs with control until your feet touch the floor.

Bent-over fly

Shoulders and upper back

- Stand with one leg in front of the other, holding a weight in each hand.
- Lean forward from your waist.
- Ensure that you keep your back flat.
- With your palms facing each other lift your arms sideways until the weights are level with your shoulders.
- Squeeze your shoulder blades while lifting.
- Lower the weights slowly.

91

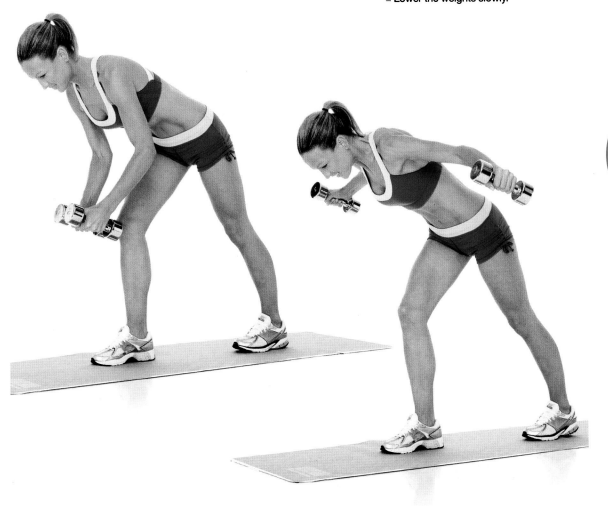

Kneeling row

Upper back

- Kneel on all fours.
- Hold a weight in your left hand and support your bodyweight on your right arm.
- Pull the weight up towards your armpit.
- Hold the top position for one second before lowering the weight.
- Don't let the weight rest on the floor.
- Repeat on the other side.

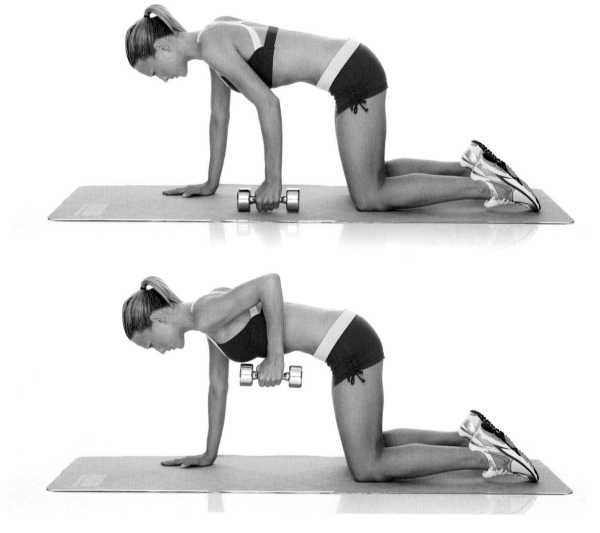

Dumbbell swing

Back, bottom, thighs and shoulders

▪ Stand holding a weight, with your feet planted firmly on the floor slightly wider than hip-width apart and with your toes pointing slightly out.
▪ Keeping your chest up and shoulders back, soften your knees and tip forwards from your hips, pushing the weight back between your knees.
▪ As the weight swings forwards, drive through your hips and swing the weight up over your head so that your arm is straight but not locked and your shoulders and hips are level.
▪ Reverse the movement and allow your body to tip as the weight swings back through your knees.
▪ At the top of the movement really focus on squeezing your bottom and keeping your shoulder blades braced back.
▪ Repeat on the other side.

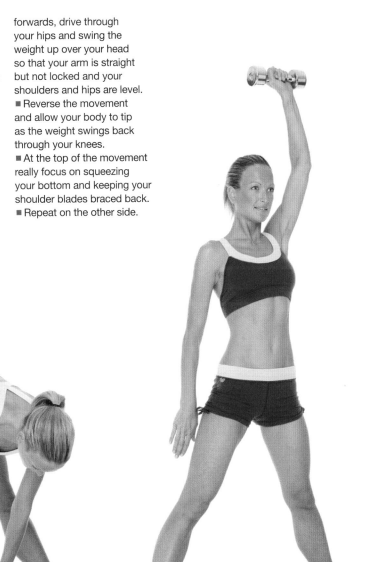

93

Back guidelines

REPS AND SETS (WEIGHTED EXERCISES):
Beginners: 2 sets of 10 to 15 repetitions using a light weight
Intermediate: 2 to 3 sets of 20 repetitions using a light weight
Advanced: 3 sets of 10 to 15 repetitions using a moderate weight

REPS AND SETS (NON-WEIGHTED EXERCISES):
Beginners: 2 sets of 10 repetitions
Intermediate: 2 sets of 20 repetitions
Advanced: 3 sets of 20 repetitions

94

About the back
According to the charity BackCare, back pain affects up to 80 per cent of the British population at some stage in their lives, and nothing is more debilitating than a bad back. Lower back pain is increasingly common among office workers, so it's important to strengthen your back. Having a strong upper back will improve your posture and help prevent slouching. Having a strong lower back will help support your stomach muscles.

For best results
■ Perform the exercises slowly. Don't speed up as this will cause you to use momentum rather than strength.
■ Never sacrifice quality for quantity.

Stomach

Lying leg extension

<u>Stomach and side muscles</u>

- Sit on the floor and lean backwards onto your elbows.
- Bend your knees to 90 degrees. This is the start position.
- Extend your legs forwards without touching the floor.
- Bend your knees to return to the start position.

Tips:
- Pull your belly button towards your spine
to prevent your back from arching.
- If you feel tension in your back, lift your feet higher off the floor.

96

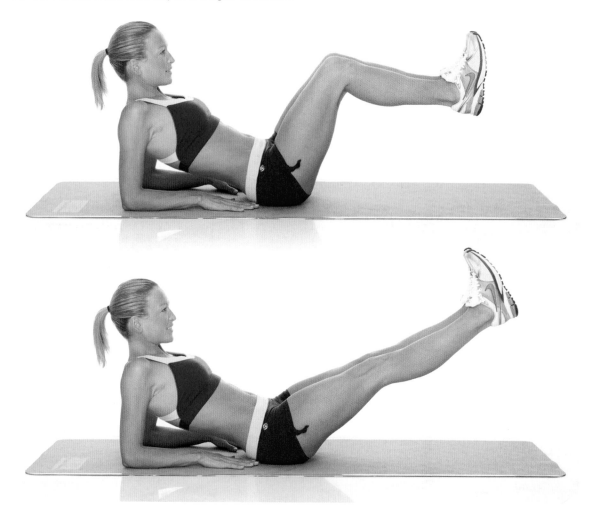

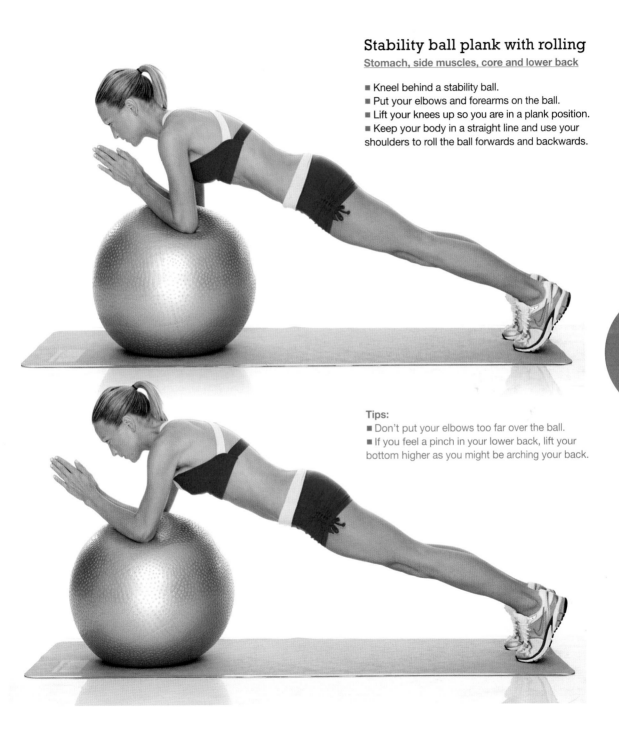

Stability ball plank with rolling

Stomach, side muscles, core and lower back

- Kneel behind a stability ball.
- Put your elbows and forearms on the ball.
- Lift your knees up so you are in a plank position.
- Keep your body in a straight line and use your shoulders to roll the ball forwards and backwards.

Tips:
- Don't put your elbows too far over the ball.
- If you feel a pinch in your lower back, lift your bottom higher as you might be arching your back.

97

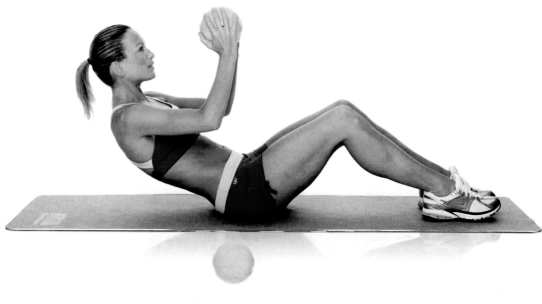

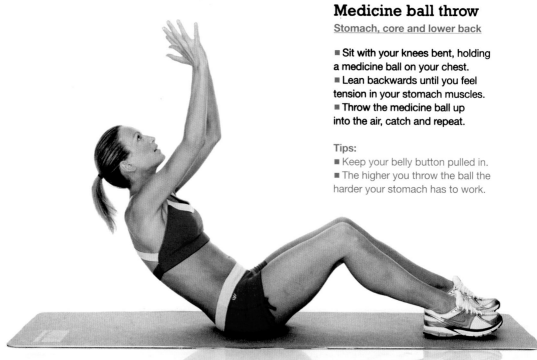

Medicine ball throw

Stomach, core and lower back

- Sit with your knees bent, holding a medicine ball on your chest.
- Lean backwards until you feel tension in your stomach muscles.
- Throw the medicine ball up into the air, catch and repeat.

Tips:
- Keep your belly button pulled in.
- The higher you throw the ball the harder your stomach has to work.

Crunches with legs at 90 degrees
<u>Stomach</u>

- Lie on your back with your legs at 90 degrees.
- Put your hands next to your temples and look up.
- Lift your shoulders two inches off
the floor, relax and repeat.

Tips:
- Don't pull your knees in towards your chest.
- Keep looking at the same point
throughout the movement.

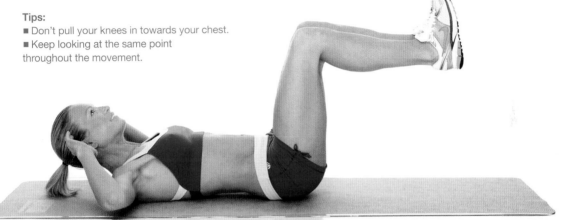

99

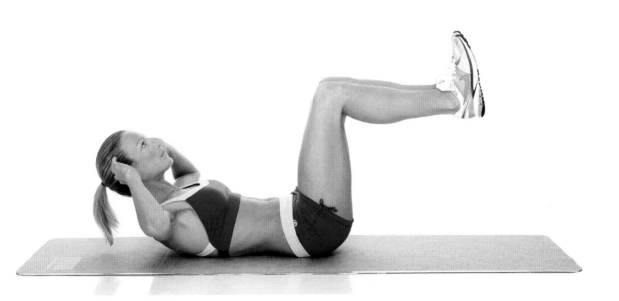

The half roll-back

<u>Stomach and core</u>

■ Sit on the floor with your heels on the floor, your knees slightly bent and your arms straight out in front of you. This is the start position.
■ Tuck your tummy in and tip your pelvis backwards so that your lower back forms a C-shape.
■ Roll back a little more so that you can roll off your sit bones on to your tailbone.
■ Pause for a couple of seconds and then return to the start position.

100

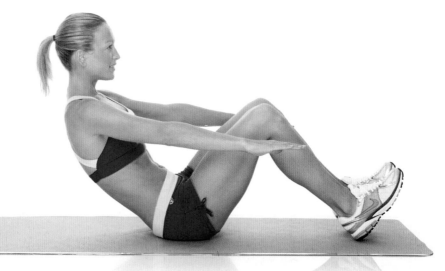

Tips:
■ Don't roll back too far; you only need to move a small amount.
■ If your tailbone feels sore, place a cushion underneath you for comfort.
■ Always return to the start position.
■ Exhale on the way back and breathe in on the way up.

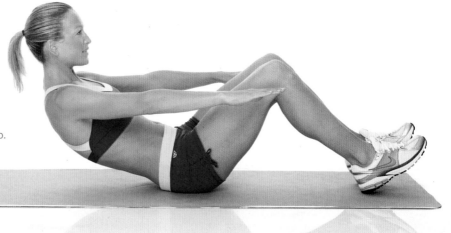

V-sits

<u>Lower stomach</u>

- Sit on the floor with your knees bent
and your arms by your sides.
- Lift both feet off the floor and start to lower your
body with your arms straight out in front of you.
- Lower your upper body further
while extending your legs.
- Lift up with control into the seated position.
- Don't let your feet touch the floor.

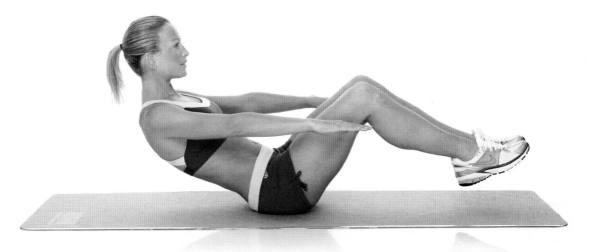

101

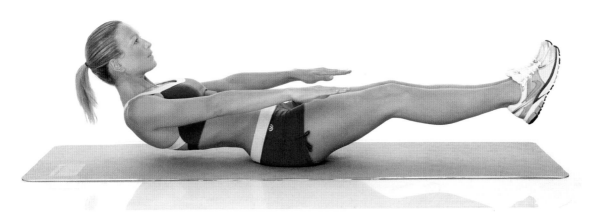

Stomach guidelines

REPS AND SETS:
Beginners: 2 sets of 10 repetitions
Intermediate: 2 sets of 15 repetitions
Advanced: 2 sets of 20 repetitions

About the stomach
You have four tummy muscles. The most commonly trained stomach muscle is your six-pack muscle (rectus abdominus), which runs from your ribcage down to your hip bones. Your side muscles (internal and external obliques) make up the next two. You have a deeper and outer layer on both sides. By training these muscles you will shape your waistline. Lastly you have your deeper abdominal muscle (transverse abdominus). This muscle is mostly trained when you do core and balancing exercises. The stomach is always a difficult area to flatten, but if you are doing regular cardiovascular work to burn calories and keeping an eye on your diet, it should be possible to flatten your tummy.

For best results
■ Perform the exercises slowly. Don't speed up as this will cause you to use momentum rather than strength.
■ Never sacrifice quality for quantity.
■ Stop and rest if you need to.

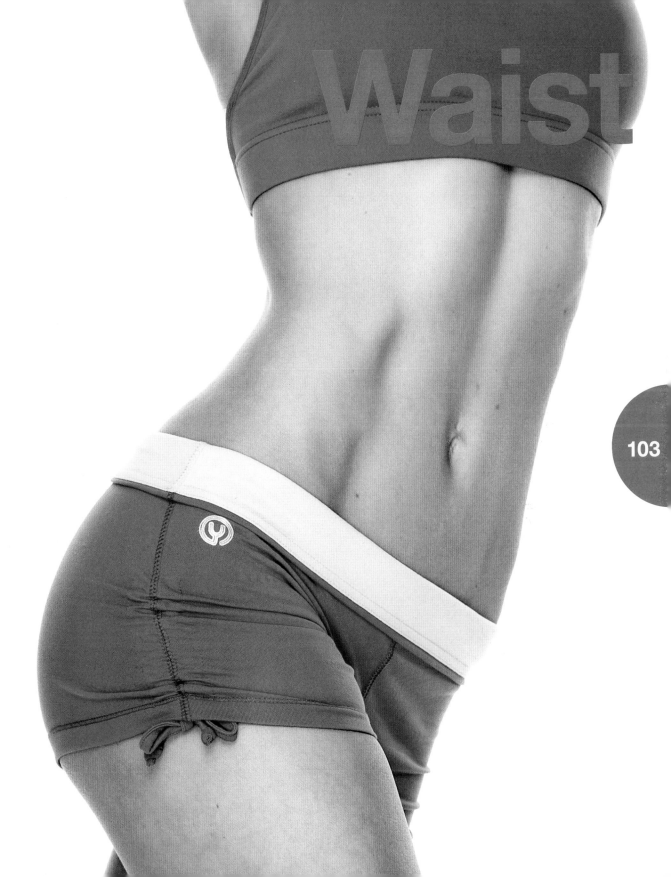

103

Dumbbell side bend

<u>Side muscles</u>

- Stand with your legs shoulder-width apart.
- Hold a weight in your left hand and hold your right hand behind your head. This is the start position.
- Bend sideways to your right side (opposite to the weight).
- Return to the start position or slightly further over towards the weight.
- Repeat on the other side.

Tip: Don't lean forwards while bending sideways.

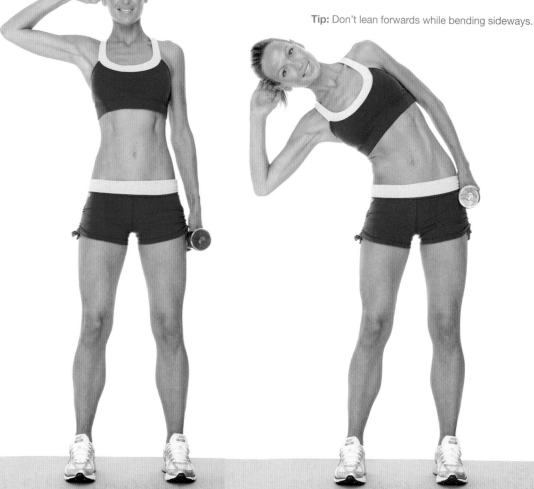

104

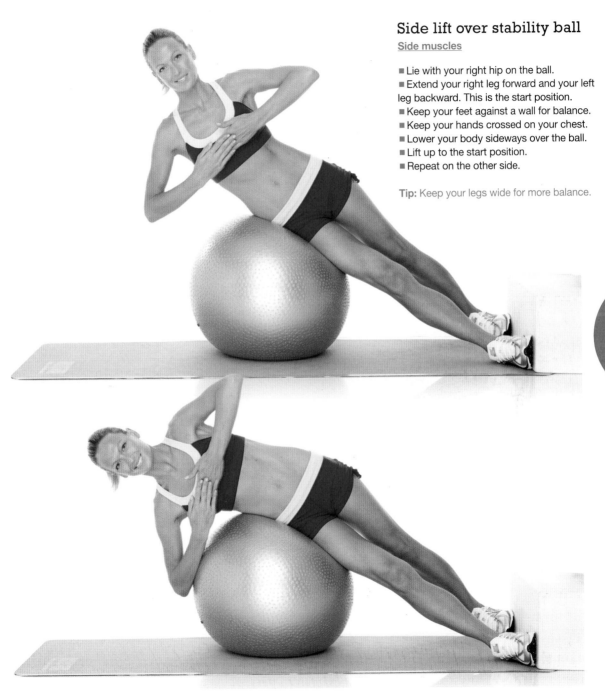

Side lift over stability ball

Side muscles

- Lie with your right hip on the ball.
- Extend your right leg forward and your left leg backward. This is the start position.
- Keep your feet against a wall for balance.
- Keep your hands crossed on your chest.
- Lower your body sideways over the ball.
- Lift up to the start position.
- Repeat on the other side.

Tip: Keep your legs wide for more balance.

105

Side leg lift

Side muscles

■ Lie on your right side in a straight line.
■ Keep your left hand on the floor for balance and support your head with your right hand.
■ Lift both legs off the floor, keeping your feet together.
■ Hold the top position for two seconds before lowering your legs.
■ Repeat on the other side.

Tip: If your hip bone hurts roll slightly forward or backward until you find a comfortable position.

106

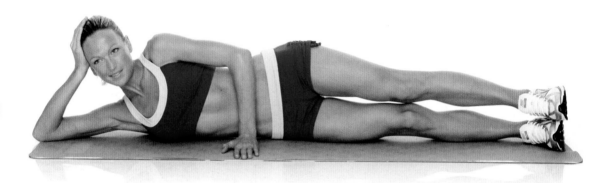

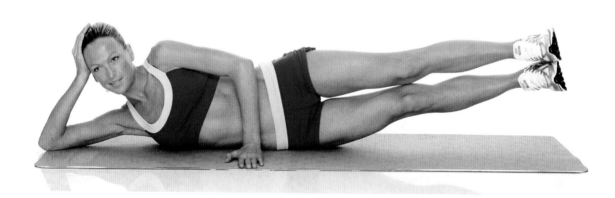

Side knee to elbow

<u>Side muscles</u>

- Lie on your right side.
- Roll slightly backwards to rest on
the soft part of your bottom.
- Keep your hands behind your head.
- Lift both legs off the floor.
- Tuck your knees in until your top
knee touches your top elbow.
- Extend your legs keeping them off the floor.
- Repeat on the other side.

Tip: Pull your belly button to
your spine to aid balance.

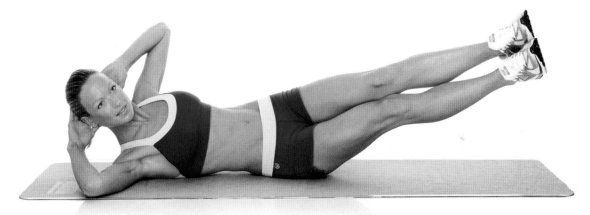

107

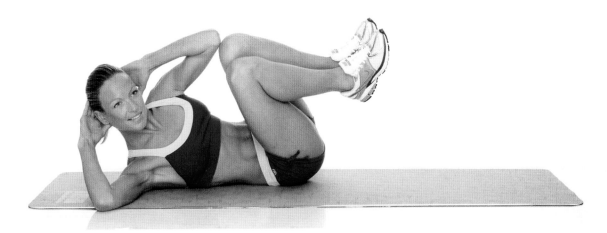

Side lying crunch

Stomach and side muscles

- Lie on your right side with your knees slightly bent.
- Put your right hand behind your head and your left hand on your left hip.
- Lift your right shoulder off the floor approximately three to four inches.
- Lower your body but try not to rest on the floor.
- Repeat on the other side.

Tip: Don't worry if you find this exercise hard, it can take a few months to master. If necessary, ask someone to hold your legs down as this will make lifting your upper body easier.

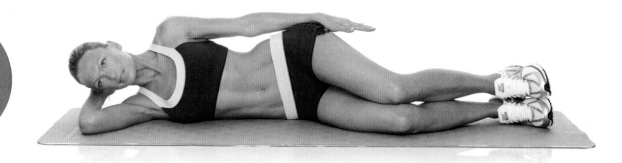

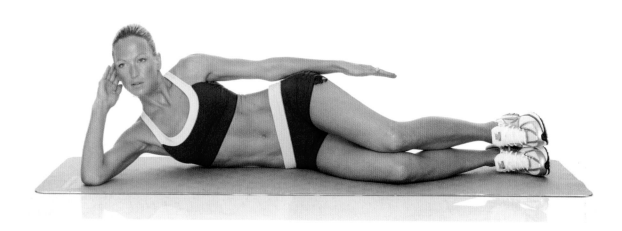

Side plank
Side muscles

■ Lie on your right side with your right elbow
directly underneath your shoulder.
■ Keep your legs straight with your feet on top of each other.
■ Lift your hips off the floor until you form a straight
line between your feet, knees, hips and shoulders.
■ Hold the position for 20 to 60 seconds on each side.
■ Repeat on the other side.

Tips:
■ If you find this too hard, keep your knees
bent and only lift your hips off the floor.
■ If you feel a lot of pressure on your supporting
shoulder, check your elbow is directly underneath your
shoulder when you are in the elevated position.

109

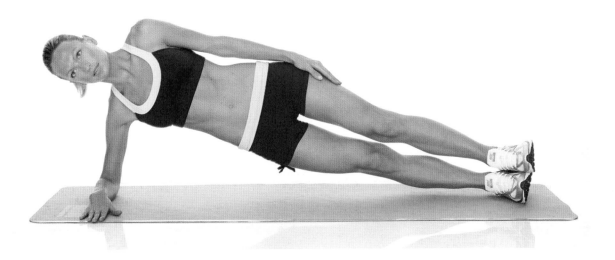

Waist guidelines

REPS AND SETS:

Beginners: 2 sets of 10 repetitions
Intermediates: 2 sets of 15 repetitions
Advanced: 2 sets of 20 repetitions
Repeat sets and reps on both the left and right side

About the waist
We all dream of a slim waistline and most of us will do anything to avoid the 'muffin-top' look, where spare flesh bulges over the top of jeans. Having a slim waist creates a feminine V-shape to the body, but more importantly, a waistline of 35 inches or more can increase your risk of heart disease and diabetes. If you tend to store excess fat around the waist then healthy eating and cardio exercise will help you lose inches off your waist, but moves to tone the waist will also help create a shapely, feminine figure.

For best results
■ Perform the exercises slowly. Don't bounce or use the body's momentum to do the exercise.
■ Never sacrifice quality for quantity.
■ Stop and rest if you need to.

110

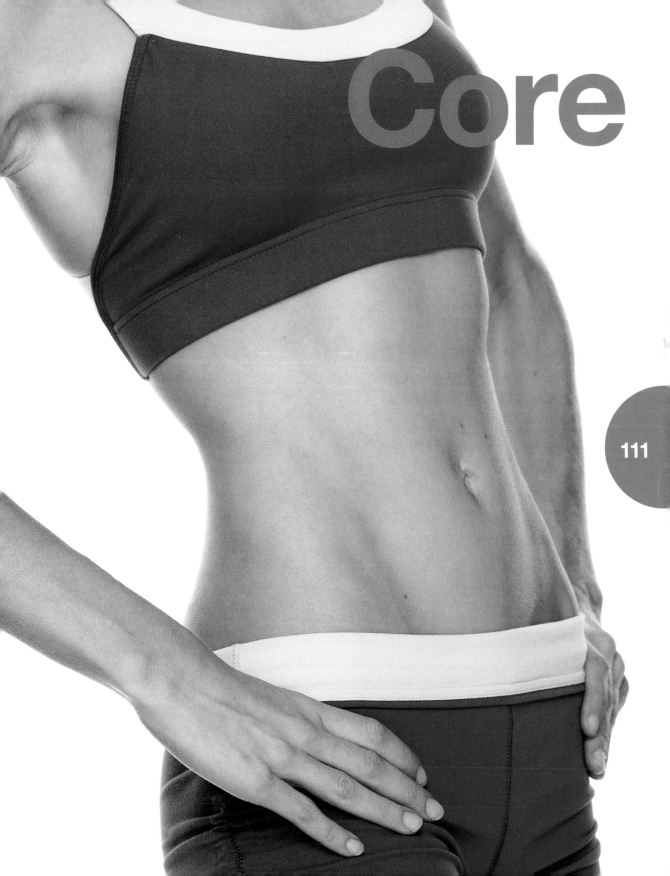

Core

111

Your powerhouse
Train your core

Having a strong core can help prevent injury and back pain, so always include core exercises in your routine

Why train the core, you might ask? In previous decades, our attitude to exercise was quite simple: burn calories with cardio, strengthen your limbs with weights,

then stretch. In recent years, however, we have realised that the core plays a huge role in injury prevention and stabilising the body. Here are some key facts about the core…

Where is the core?
When people talk about the core, the area they are predominantly referring to is the midsection/stomach or back, i.e. the area of your body that would be covered if you were wearing a corset. But, to be more specific, the core is in the area of our lumbar spine and pelvis and incorporates our deep spinal, abdominal and pelvic muscles. These are muscles such as the transverse abdominus (which run from our sides to our front), the multifidus (positioned deep in the spine), the obliques (the sides of the stomach), the gluteus medius/minimus (bottom) and the pelvic floor.

What does it help us do?
Our core provides the body with stability and support before and during movement. The core will assist in giving the upper and lower body a better platform from which to move. The core helps us maximise force generation and minimise joint loads in all types of activity. For example, when pulling or pushing we require some core strength to keep the body upright.

Why do we need to train it?
Training your core helps minimise the risk of injury to your upper and lower body and back. Training core muscles can be beneficial in maintaining back and pelvis stability and allows the more superficial muscles that produce movement to do their job.

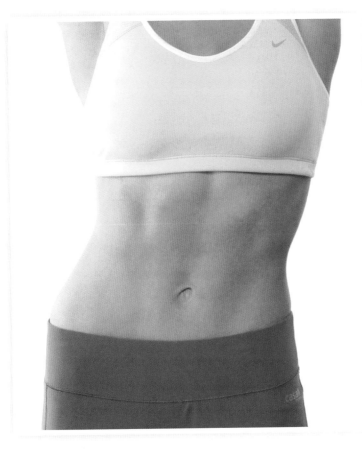

'Our core provides the body
with stability and support
before and during movement'

What happens if the core is weak?
If our core muscles are weak or not
activating efficiently, stress on joints
such as our lumbar vertebrae (towards
the base of the spine), shoulders and
knees is increased. A weak core causes
an increase in muscle activation of
other muscle groups, which causes
poor movement patterns (wrong
muscles doing the work), which could
lead to injury. For example, when
running you can stress the back and
knee joints if your bottom and back
muscles are not working well.

**What are the benefits of having
a strong core?**
A strong core allows us to use the
power muscles we have and when
we move we will be able to do so with
greater efficiency, economy and power.
A strong core also supports the spine.

**What common myths are associated
with training the core?**
It is a myth that sit-ups train the core, as
the six-pack (rectus abdominals) are not
our core muscles; they are the superficial
muscles or prime movers of our trunk.
Also, many people assume that we just
have to pull in our belly button or suck
up through our pelvic floor to strengthen
our core. Pulling in our stomach will
activate the core initially, but once we
can move efficiently with good stability
there is no need to keep 'drawing in' or
'switching on' our core. Core muscles

are our deep stabilisers and their role is
to provide support in sitting, standing
or movement and should be activated
without us even being aware of it.

**What are the best ways to train
the core?**
It is important to find the level you are
at with your core and pelvis stability
and then find out the appropriate
exercises. Many of us do core exercises
that are too hard for us, which means
we continue to move using the wrong
muscle groups. Sometimes it is
better to move with ease rather than
tightening everything up. Also, make
your exercise progress functional,
using a range of movements or ones
that are specific to your sport.

**How often should we train the
core for best results?**
Our core muscles are deep, stabilising
muscles that are designed to work for
long periods so we should exercise
daily to try to improve them.

**Are there any easy ways we can
train the core?**
Yes, very slightly pulling your belly
button towards your spine can help if
you have never done core exercises
before, as this is a simple way of
getting your core muscles working.
Sitting upright will also help, as to
maintain this position you will activate
your deep stability muscles.

Key facts about the core

- Core muscles are
obliques (sides of the
stomach), abdominals
(stomach), lower back and
the glutes (bottom).
- The core muscles are
often called the 'power
zone' or 'powerhouse' of
the body.
- Having a strong core
can decrease or prevent
injuries that are linked with
back pain.
- Having a strong core can
also improve posture.
- Pilates is ideal for
strengthening the core.

113

If you follow the exercises on the
next four pages, you will be able
to strengthen your core, which will
help you move more efficiently
and prevent the risk of injury.

Core engage

Core

■ Lie on your back with your knees bent and your feet flat.
■ Roll your pelvis back and forth until you find a midpoint where your back is neither pushed into the floor nor arched excessively.
■ Keeping your shoulders relaxed and drawn down, place your fingertips palm down underneath your lower back.
■ Take a breath in, allowing your abdominal wall to expand outwards.

■ As you exhale, draw the navel inwards and slowly lift your right foot until your knee is above your hip.
■ Breathe in and slowly lower your foot back to the floor.
■ Relax and repeat with your left leg.

Tips:
■ There should be no change in pressure on your fingertips between your back.
■ Try to stay relaxed throughout the exercise and try not to hunch your shoulders.

114

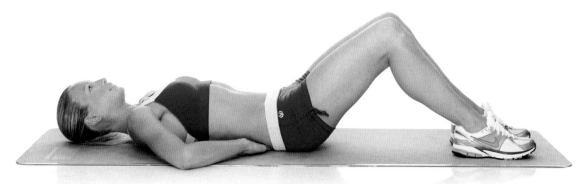

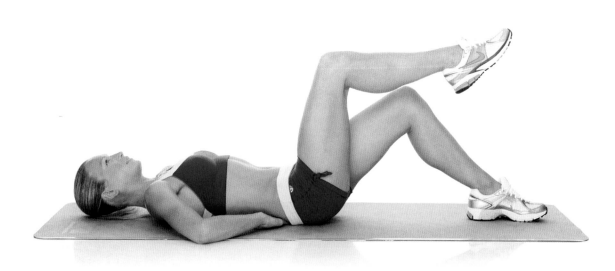

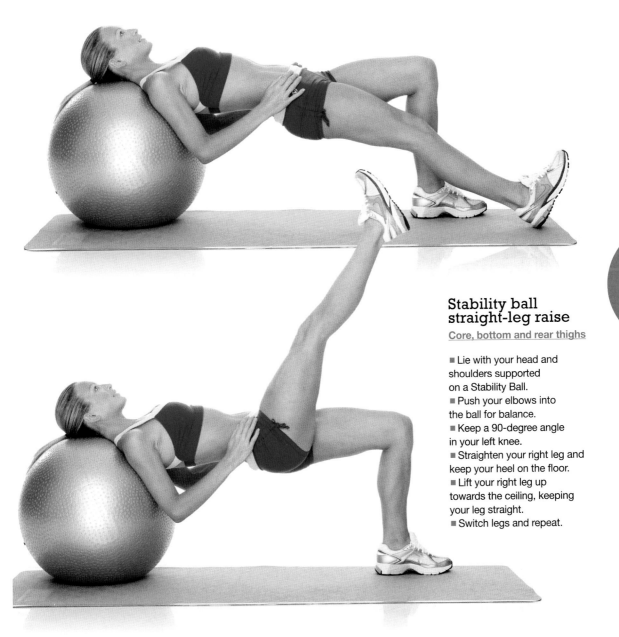

Stability ball straight-leg raise

Core, bottom and rear thighs

■ Lie with your head and shoulders supported on a Stability Ball.
■ Push your elbows into the ball for balance.
■ Keep a 90-degree angle in your left knee.
■ Straighten your right leg and keep your heel on the floor.
■ Lift your right leg up towards the ceiling, keeping your leg straight.
■ Switch legs and repeat.

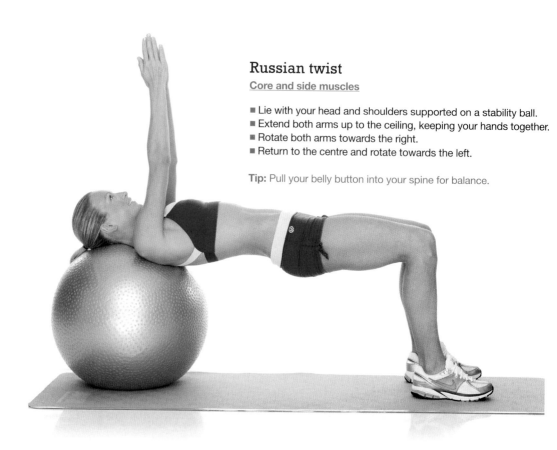

Russian twist

<u>Core and side muscles</u>

- Lie with your head and shoulders supported on a stability ball.
- Extend both arms up to the ceiling, keeping your hands together.
- Rotate both arms towards the right.
- Return to the centre and rotate towards the left.

Tip: Pull your belly button into your spine for balance.

116

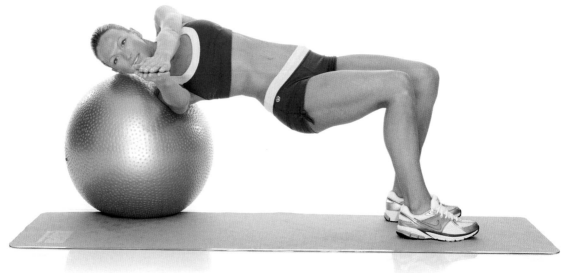

Kneeling on stability ball
Core, legs and arms

- Stand behind the stability ball.
- Lean forward and place your hands and knees hip-width apart on the stability ball.
- Roll slowly forward to lift your feet off the floor.
- Hold the all fours position.
- Hold the position twice for 20 seconds.

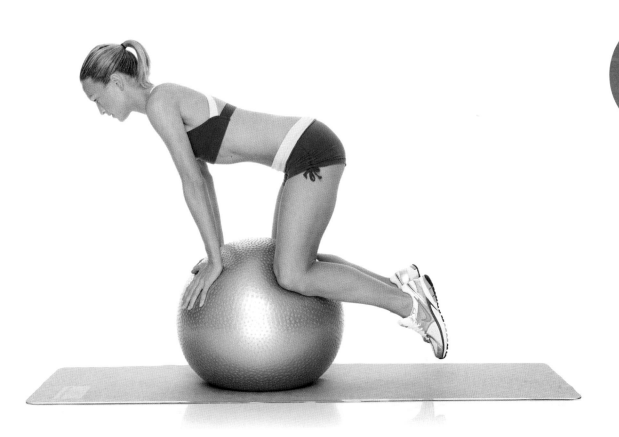

Core guidelines

REPS AND SETS:
Beginners: 2 sets of 10 reps
Intermediates: 2 sets of 15 reps
Advanced: 2 sets of 20 reps

About the core
In basic terms, the core is the torso of the body – if you were to take away your arms and legs all you would have left would be the core. The core incorporates our deep spinal, abdominal and pelvic muscles. These are muscles such as the transverse abdominus (deeper stomach muscles), multifidus (muscles along the vertebral column), obliques (side muscles), gluteus medius/minimus (bottom), pelvic floor and the diaphragm. Having a strong core can decrease or alleviate back pain too.

For best results
- Aim to exercise your core daily. Simply pulling your belly button into your spine will achieve this.
- Breathe normally when working the core.
- Pilates can also help strengthen the core.

118

Fat burners

Dumbbell walking lunges

Thighs and bottom

■ Stand with feet hip-width apart, holding a pair of dumbbells in your hands, palms facing your sides.
■ Take a large step forward bending both knees to 90 degrees.
■ Push through your front foot, activating your bottom to go into the next step. Continue alternating legs with each rep till you complete the set.

Tip:
■ Don't let your front knee go over your toes.

Weights
Beginners 4-6kg in each hand
Intermediate 6-10kg in each hand
Advanced 12kg in each hand

120

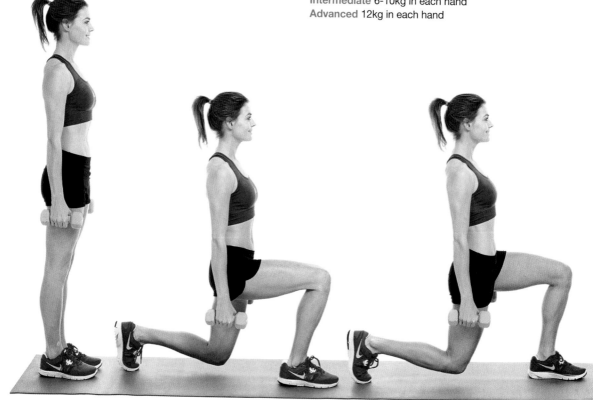

Dumbbell split squats
Thighs and bottom

■ Stand with your feet hip-width apart, holding a pair of dumbbells in your hands, palms facing your sides.
■ Raise one foot so it's resting on a bench behind you. Position your front foot in the lunge position in front of you.
■ Keeping your back straight, lower your body into a lunge, placing your weight on the front leg. Return to the start position and repeat to complete one set before repeating on the other leg.

Tip:
■ Ensure the back leg keeps a slight bend.

Weights
Beginners 4-6kg in each hand
Intermediate 6-10kg in each hand
Advanced 12kg in each hand

121

Dumbbell lunge jumps

<u>Thighs and bottom</u>

■ Stand with your feet hip-width apart, holding a pair of dumbbells in your hands, palms facing your sides.
■ Step one foot forward and lower down into a lunge, making sure your front knee doesn't go over your toes.
■ Jump up and change your legs in mid-air.

■ Land softly and go straight into another lunge with the other foot forward. Repeat and switch legs with every rep to complete set.

Weights
Beginners body weight or 2kg in each hand
Intermediate 4-6kg in each hand
Advanced 8kg in each hand

122

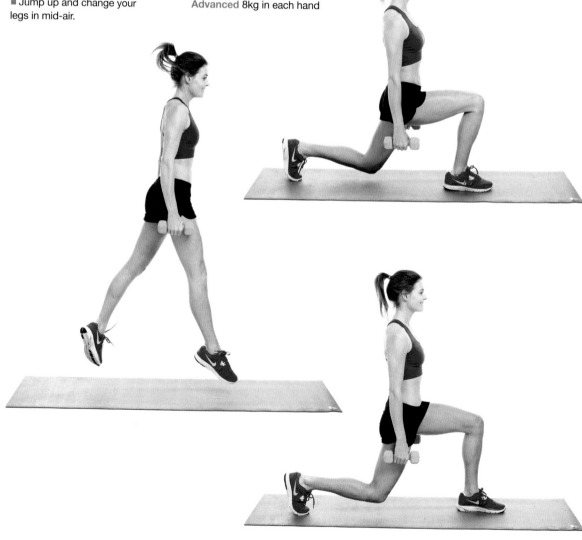

Stability ball hamstring curls

Bottom and back of thighs

■ Lie on your back with your feet on the ball.
■ Raise your hips and drag the ball in towards you.
■ As the ball comes in, continue to raise your hips so you finish each rep on your shoulders with your legs bent. Repeat to complete set.

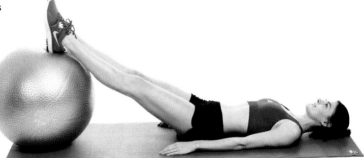

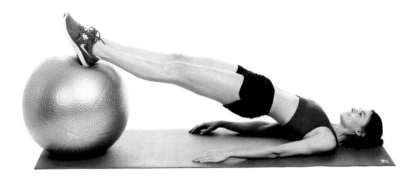

123

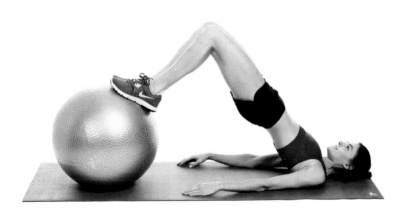

Stability ball knee tucks
<u>Core and shoulders</u>

■ Begin with your arms in the press-up position, with your feet resting on top of a stability ball.
■ Keeping your core activated, bring the ball in toward your arms, keeping your lower back parallel to the floor throughout each rep.
■ Repeat to complete set.

124

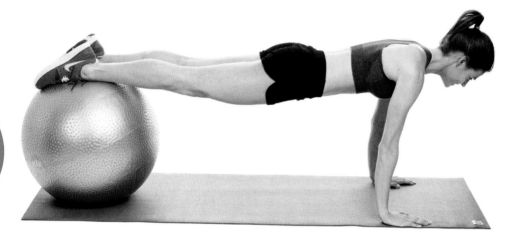

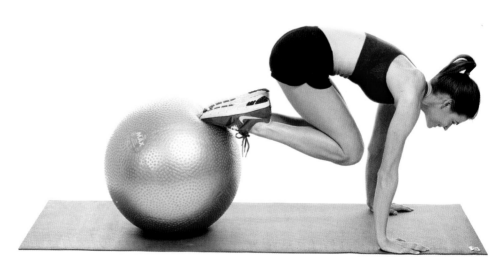

Stability ball elbow roll-outs

<u>Core and lower stomach</u>

■ Adopt the plank position on a stability ball: shoulders over elbows, body in a straight line, legs straight out behind you.
■ Push the ball forward and back using your arms. Make sure the rest of your body remains still throughout each rep.
■ Repeat to complete set.

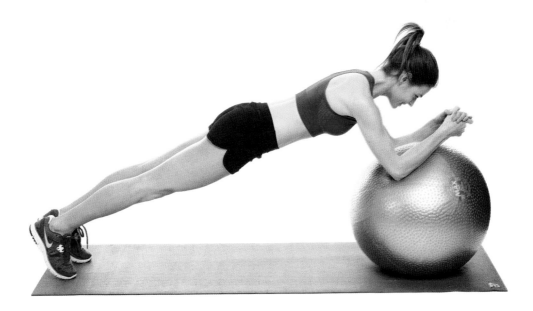

125

Body weight leg drops

Lower stomach

- Lie on your back, then raise your legs to the ceiling.
- Lower your legs to the floor, keeping your core engaged.
- Return to the start position and repeat to complete set.

Tip:
- Keep your knees slightly bent throughout each rep.

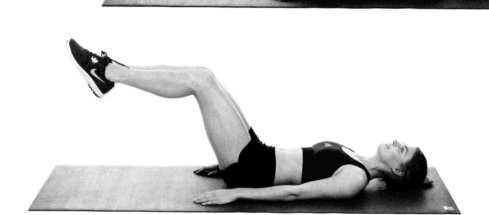

126

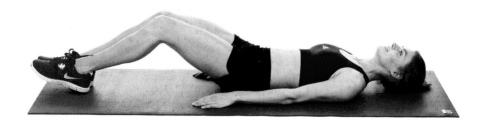

Plank elbow raises
Core and side muscles

■ Begin in the plank position: shoulders over elbows, body in a straight line, legs straight out behind you.
■ While keeping your body in the same position, raise one arm out to 90 degrees to the side, activating your core.
■ Only raise your arm till it's parallel to the floor before returning to the start position and repeating with the other arm.
■ Continue alternating arms to complete set.

127

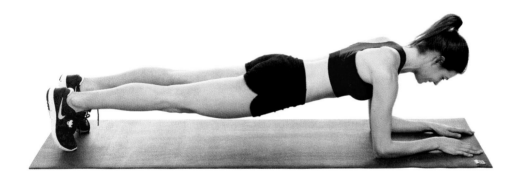

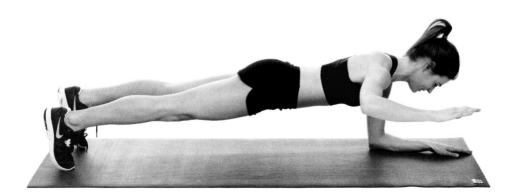

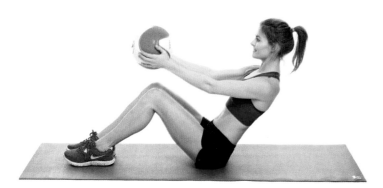

Medicine ball rotations

Side muscles and lower stomach

- Sit on the floor with your knees slightly bent and your back straight.
- Hold a medicine ball in front of you with both hands.
- Lean back to 45 degrees then rotate from side to side, touching the floor with the medicine ball.
- Continue alternating sides to complete set.

Weights

Beginners 2-4kg
Intermediate 4-6kg
Advanced 8kg

128

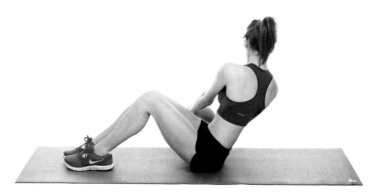

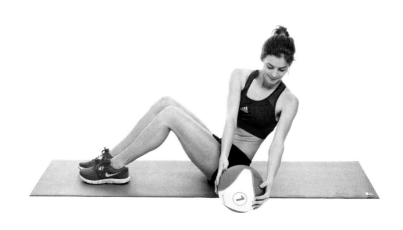

Medicine ball sit-up raises

Stomach, arms and shoulders

- Lie flat on your back holding
a medicine ball over your chest.
- Sit up, straightening your arms and
raising the medicine ball above your head.
- Return to the start position before repeating
to complete the set.

Weights
Beginners 4-6kg
Intermediate 6-10kg
Advanced 12kg

129

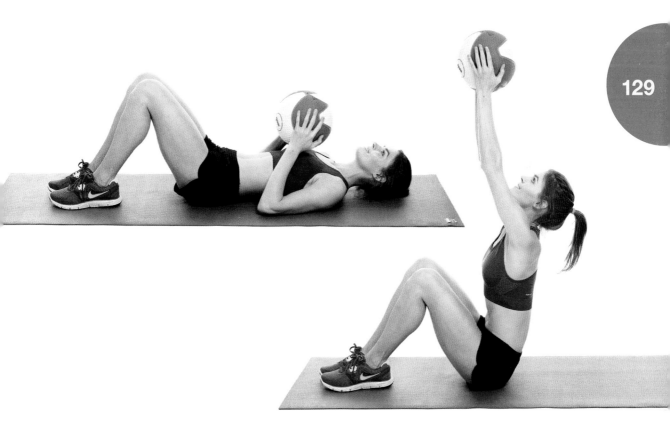

Press-up shoulder tap

Chest, shoulders, rear of upper arms and core

■ Begin in the press-up position: shoulders over hands, your body in a straight line from shoulders to ankles.
■ Lower down into a full press-up.
■ Push back up and tap your right hand on your left shoulder. Repeat, making sure you change hands each time to complete set.

130

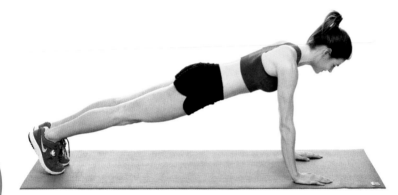

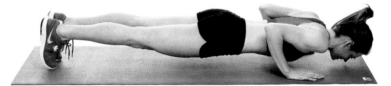

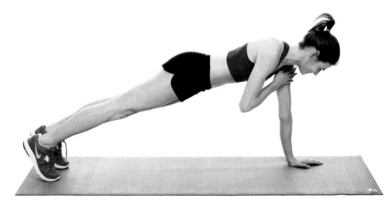

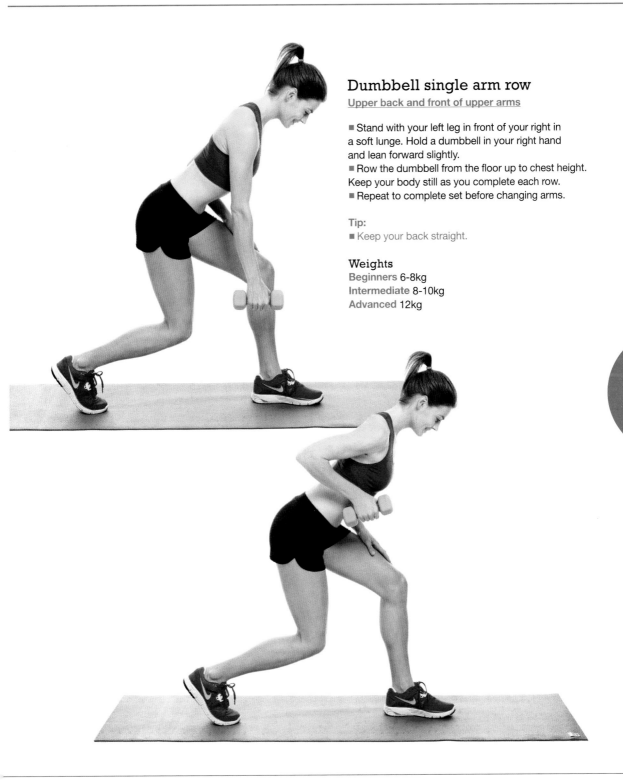

Dumbbell single arm row
Upper back and front of upper arms

■ Stand with your left leg in front of your right in a soft lunge. Hold a dumbbell in your right hand and lean forward slightly.
■ Row the dumbbell from the floor up to chest height. Keep your body still as you complete each row.
■ Repeat to complete set before changing arms.

Tip:
■ Keep your back straight.

Weights
Beginners 6-8kg
Intermediate 8-10kg
Advanced 12kg

131

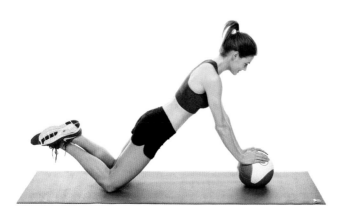

Medicine ball explosive press-up

Chest, shoulders, rear of upper arms and core

■ Rest your knees on the floor and grip a medicine ball with both hands. Using this close grip, lower your chest down toward your hands.
■ On the way up from each rep, push hard off the ball and land with your hands on either side of the ball.
■ From this wider position perform another press-up, then push up again, landing both hands on the ball (the original position). Continue to swap the position of your hands with each rep.

132

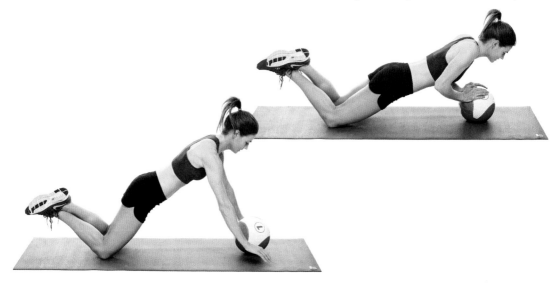

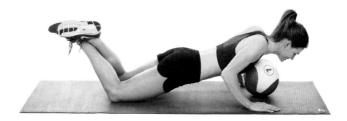

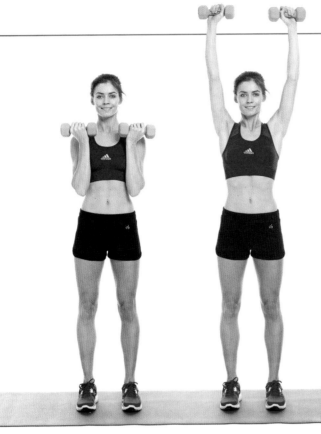

Dumbbell shoulder turn and press
Shoulders and chest

- Stand with your feet shoulder-width apart.
- Hold a pair of dumbbells, palms facing in, at your shoulders.
- Press the dumbbells up towards the ceiling. Make sure you turn the dumbbells with each rep so your palms end up facing away from you with each rep.
- Repeat to complete set.

Weights
Beginners 4-6kg in each hand
Intermediate 6-8kg in each hand
Advanced 8kg in each hand

133

Dumbbell prone rows
Upper back and front of upper arms

- Adjust a bench to 45 degrees and lie with your chest over it.
- Make sure your head is clear of the top.
- Keeping your shoulders back, row the dumbbells up toward your armpits before slowly lowering them down.
- Repeat to complete set.

Weights
Beginners 4-6kg in each hand
Intermediate 8-10kg in each hand
Advanced 12kg in each hand

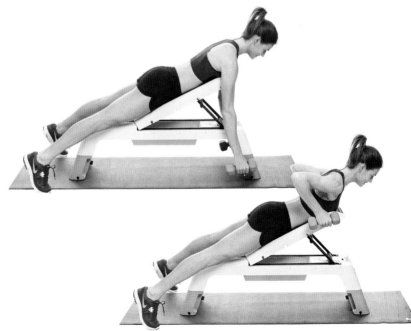

Fat-burning guidelines

REPS AND SETS (non-weighted exercises):
There are 15 fat-burning exercises which will work your upper body, lower body and core. Aim to work the entire body evenly by choosing the same number of exercises for each area.

Beginners: Choose 3-6 exercises; perform 2-3 sets of 6-8 reps.
Aim to complete this workout 1-3 times per week

Intermediate: Choose 3-6 exercises; perform 4-5 sets of 6-8 reps.
Aim to complete this workout 2-4 times per week

Advanced: Choose 3-6 exercises; perform 5-6 sets of 6-8 reps.
Aim to complete this workout 3-5 times per week

REPS AND SETS (weighted exercises):
For all levels follow the reps and sets guidelines above and see individual exercises for weights guidelines.

For best results
- Be sure to change the combination of exercises you do every six weeks to avoid your body plateauing.
- Never sacrifice quality for quantity.

134

Stretching

Lunging hip flexor stretch

Hips

- Kneel on your left knee and place your right leg in front of you.
- Place both hands on your right leg.
- Push your hips forward and pull your shoulders back.
- Hold for 30 seconds, relax and repeat on the other side.

Guidelines for stretching

It is important to stretch after exercise as it can prevent muscle soreness and improve flexibility. Be sure to always stretch while your muscles are still warm from your workout.

136

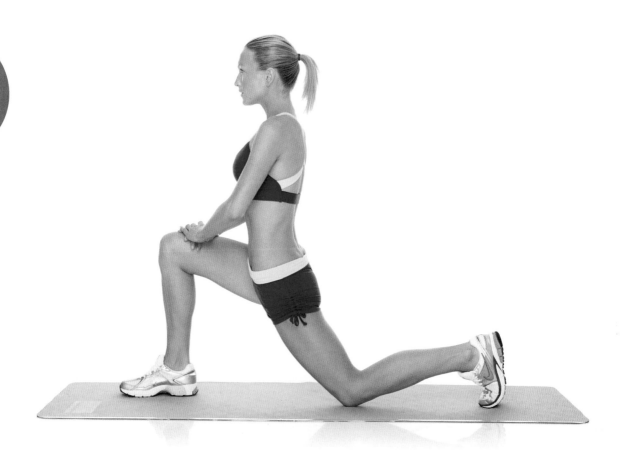

Quad stretch

<u>Front thighs</u>

■ Stand up straight with
your feet together and your
left hand on your hip.
■ Bend your right knee behind
you and hold your foot with your
right hand, pushing your foot
up towards your bottom.
■ Hold for 30 seconds, relax
and repeat on the other side.

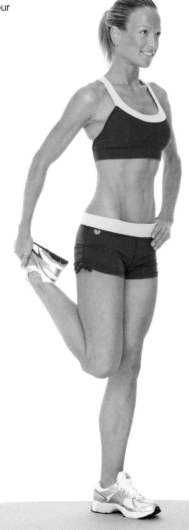

137

Wall chest stretch

<u>Chest</u>

■ Stand with your right shoulder facing a wall and place your left hand on your hip.
■ Lift your right arm and place your palm on the wall level with your head.
■ Rotate your body away from the wall to increase the stretch.
■ Hold for 30 seconds, relax and repeat on the other side.

138

Hamstring stretch

Rear thighs

■ Lie on your back with your
left leg bent and your right leg
extended up to the ceiling.
■ Grab hold of your right leg
where you feel comfortable.
■ Pull your right leg towards you.
■ Hold for 30 seconds, relax
and repeat on the other side.

Tip: The more flexible you are,
the straighter your leg will be.

139

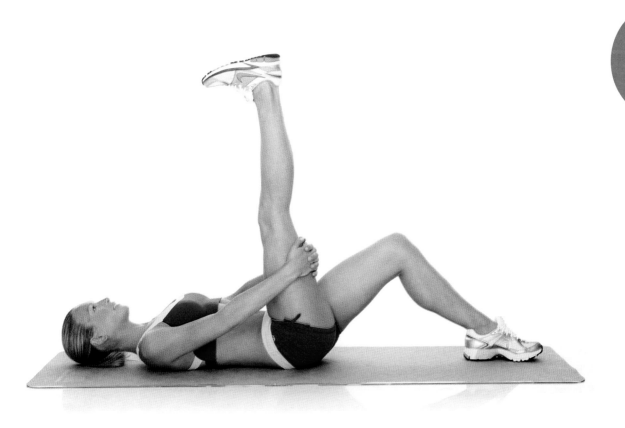

Cat stretch

<u>Back</u>

- Kneel on all fours.
- Ensure that your hands are directly underneath your shoulders and your knees are underneath your hips.
- Curl your back up to the ceiling, looking down to your knees.
- Slowly lower your back until you form a curved back.
- Do 2 sets of 10 repetitions holding each position for 2 seconds.

Tip: Never work through pain.

140

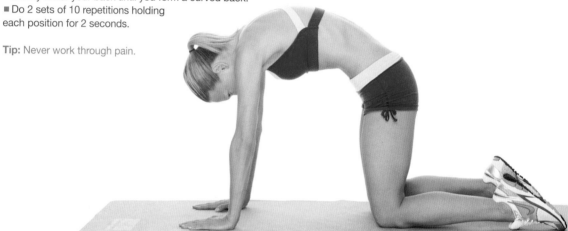

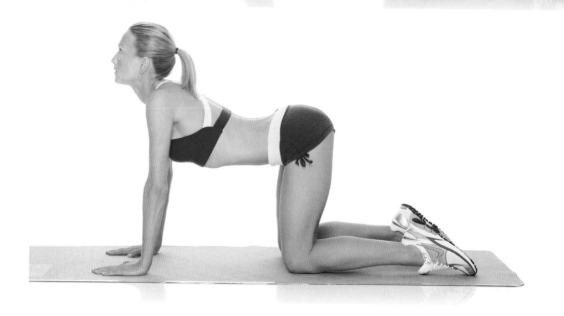

Shoulder stretch
Shoulders, arms and upper back

■ Stand facing a wall and place both palms at shoulder-height on the wall.
■ Walk your legs backwards until you feel a stretch around your shoulders, arms and back.
■ Hold for 30 seconds, then relax.

Tip: If the back of your legs are tight, you may feel a stretch all the way down to your ankles.

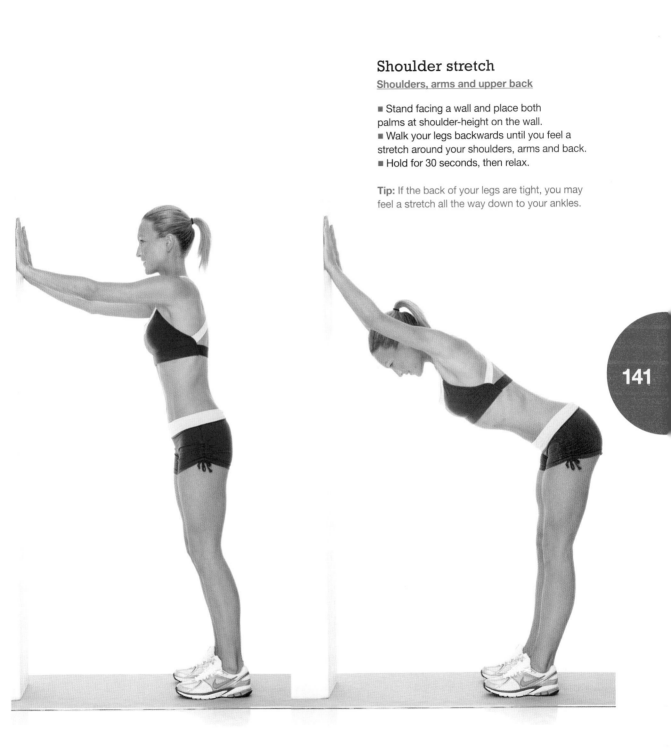

141

Glute stretch

Bottom

■ Lie face down on the floor.
■ Lift your upper body and support your head and shoulders with your arms.
■ Tuck your right leg underneath your body by placing your right foot to the left of your left knee.
■ The top of your right foot should be flat along the ground.

■ Sit back and slide your left foot backwards, keeping your right foot where it is until the front of your left leg is along the ground.
■ You should now feel a stretch in the right side of your bottom.
■ Hold for 30 seconds, relax and repeat on the other side.

Tip: Move slowly into this stretch and wiggle your hips slightly to the left or right to feel the stretch in the tightest part of your bottom.

142

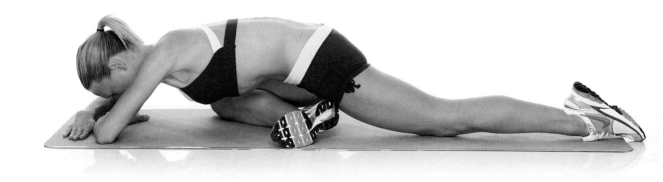

Adductor stretch

<u>Inner thighs</u>

■ Sit on the floor with your knees bent,
the soles of your feet together and your
hands resting on your ankles.
■ Allow your knees to fall out slowly to the sides.
■ You should feel a gentle stretch on your inner
thighs. If not, increase the stretch gently by pressing
your forearms down along your inner thighs.
■ Hold for 30 seconds then relax.

Tip: Keep your body upright throughout the stretch
and avoid slouching and hunching forwards.

143

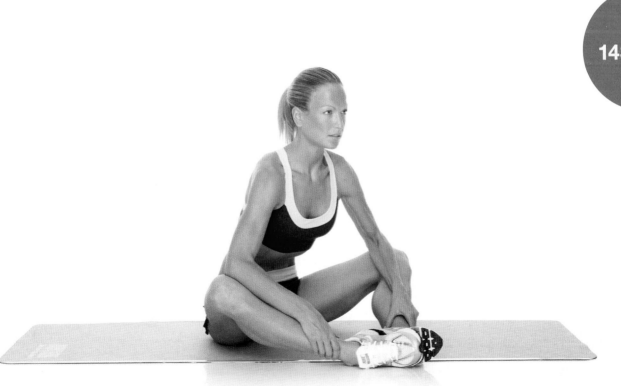

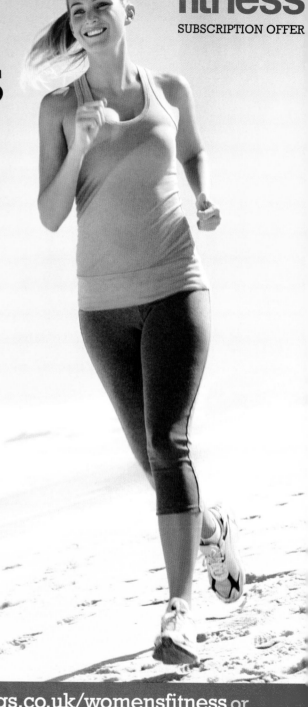
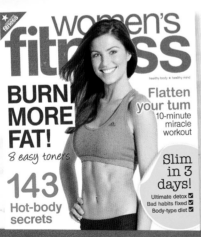

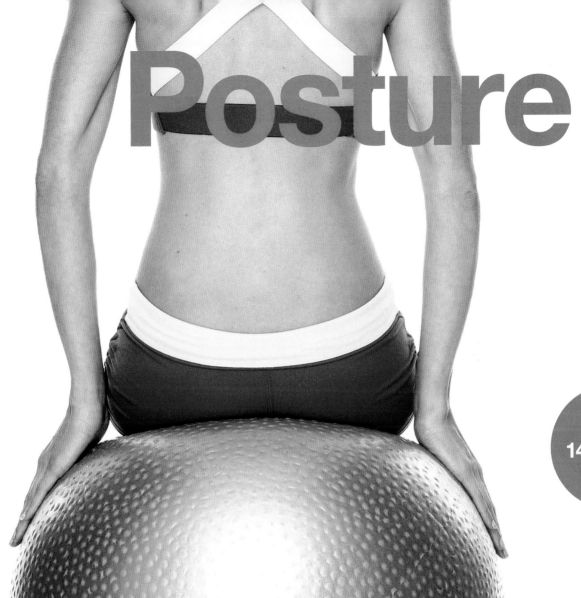

Posture

Four-point abdominal brace

Core and pelvic floor

■ Kneel on all fours.
■ Keep your spine in a neutral position, so that it is neither arched nor rounded.
■ Breathe in and allow your stomach to push out without changing your position.
■ Slowly exhale and draw your stomach in, sucking it tight as if you are trying to make your belly button touch your spine. Do this without changing position.
■ Keep exhaling and drawing the stomach in, and slowly repeat.

Tips:
■ Make sure that your hands are below your shoulders with the elbows soft and your knees directly below your hips.
■ As you draw your stomach in and exhale, try not to round your back.

146

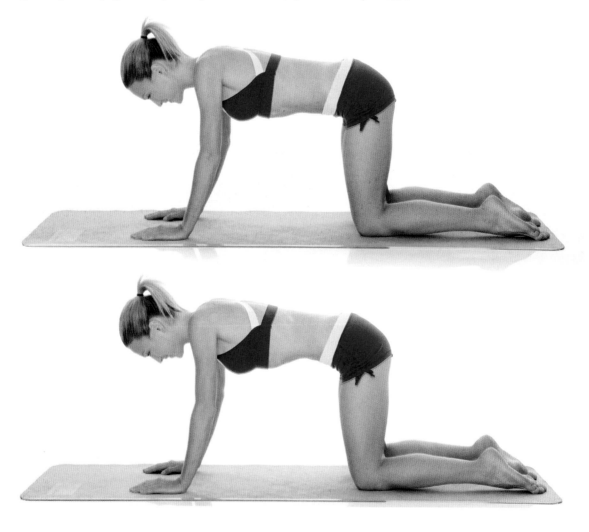

Core rotation

Waist and side muscles

■ Lie flat on your back with your spine in a neutral position.
■ Place your arms by your sides.
■ Lift your legs so that your knees are above the hips at a 90-degree angle.
■ Slowly rotate to the left, lowering the knees and hips.
■ Brace and pull back to the centre.
■ Repeat the exercise, alternating sides.

Tips:
■ Try not to elevate your shoulders or lift your head.
■ Breathe in as you lower the legs and exhale as you lift.

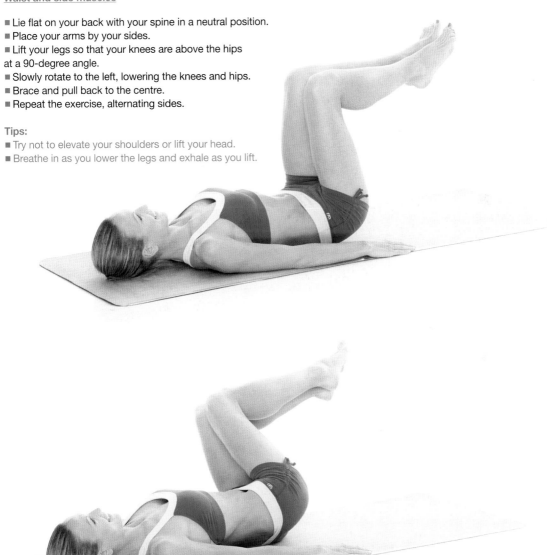

147

Braced doorway stretch

<u>Chest and shoulders</u>

- Stand in the middle of an open doorway with your feet shoulder-width apart.
- Place your right forearm and hand flat against the side of the doorframe.

- Step forwards slightly with your right foot until you feel a stretch through your chest and the front of your shoulder.
- Hold the stretch for 20 to 30 seconds and repeat on the other side.

Tip: Try not to arch your lower back.

148

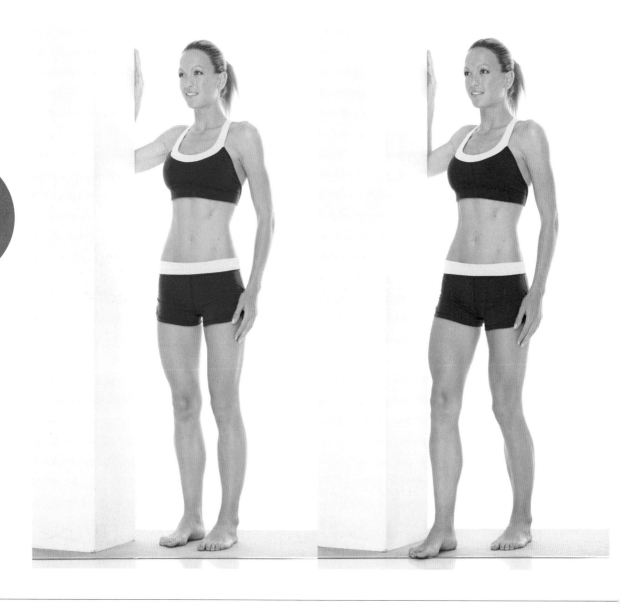

Abdominal bridge
Core and pelvic floor

- Lie face down on the floor.
- Bring your elbows underneath your shoulders and depress the shoulder girdle.
- As you exhale, suck your stomach in tight and lift your hips from the floor until they are almost the same height as your shoulders.
- Hold this position and keep breathing.

Tips:
- Go through the process slowly. As you pull your stomach in just before you lift, you should feel your stomach tighten.
- Try not to shrug your shoulders. Keep them drawn back and down to make your stomach muscles work harder.

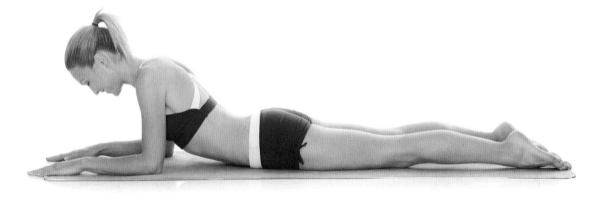

149

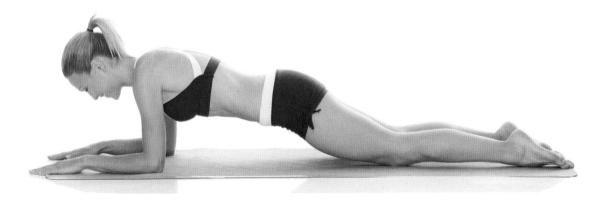

Lat to cobra stretch

<u>Upper back, stomach, hips and chest</u>

- Kneel down on the floor.
- Sit your hips back onto your heels and allow your torso to tip forwards.
- Keeping your bottom on your heels, reach forward with your hands and allow your forehead to rest on the floor.
- Walk your hands back in beneath your shoulders.
- Slide your hands forward slightly, lift your hips forwards and position them on the floor so that your chest is lifted and your shoulders are drawn back.
- Alternate between these two positions, holding each position for 20 to 30 seconds.

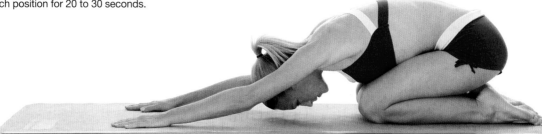

150

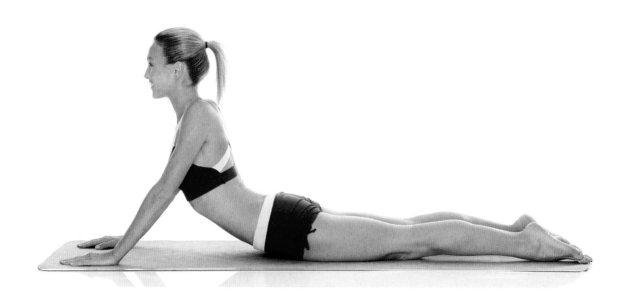

Supine glute bridge

Lower back, bottom and rear thighs

■ Lie flat on your back with your arms by your sides.
■ Bend your knees, keeping your feet flat on the floor.
■ Push your hips up into the air so that they act as a midpoint for a straight line between your knees and shoulders.

■ Slowly straighten your right leg keeping your knees together.
■ Bring your right foot back to its original position on the floor and repeat on the other side.

Tips:
■ Don't let your hips drop when you take your foot off the floor.
■ Remember to breathe.

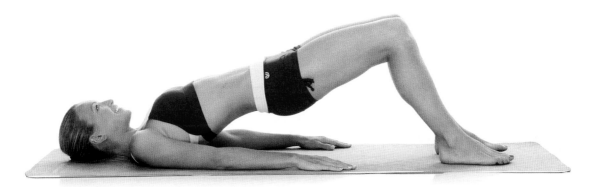

151

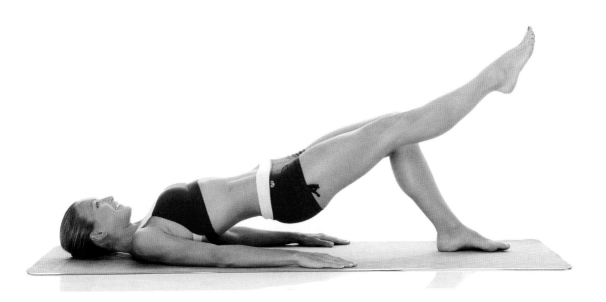

Rest to replenish
Sleep for recovery

Rest is vital for exercise recovery, but a good night's sleep isn't just about the number of hours you get, it's about quality too

We all do our best to keep as healthy as possible these days, and why shouldn't we? We only get one body and we can't trade it in for a newer model if it starts being unreliable. There's plenty of information about eating the right foods and exercising regularly to keep fit and healthy, but what about sleep? How much should we be getting, and is its quality important? And even more importantly, can it affect our overall health?

How much sleep is enough?
Let's look at our ancestors' sleeping patterns. Sleep was largely linked to when the sun rose and set due to the availability of light, which means our ancestors would have had a greater amount of sleep in the winter than in the summer. Since we're no different from people who lived 10,000 years ago, we should take note of this. SAD (Seasonal Affective Disorder) is a fairly modern development and could be linked to our lack of connection with our natural circadian rhythm (24-hour sleep/wake cycle).

We should also consider why we sleep, and what happens to our body while we sleep. Think of the body as a bank account from which we make a withdrawal when we are awake, active and alert, and which we pay back into when we sleep, as the body is able to repair itself during this time. Our immune system is just one of the systems that undergoes important repair during sleep. Ageing and degeneration will also be accelerated by lack of sleep. So if you're active and alert and making withdrawals more than you're resting and repairing and making deposits then you'll end up with a sleep debt.

Our 24-hour sleep/wake cycle is set within the first few weeks of our lives. However, with the introduction of electric light around 1880 we have been able to disrupt this cycle, and the increased use of TVs and computers has accelerated this. The light emitted from these appliances stimulates our 'wake up' hormones and reduces the production of the ones that make us sleepy.

When is the best time to sleep?
Our bodies are programmed to undergo physical repair between the hours of 10pm and 2am. Our cells divide and repair the damage of the day and if we're exercising to build up stronger muscles this is the time when the rebuilding happens. The stimulation may occur when you're working out in the gym or running in the park, but the crucial building process occurs between the hours of 10pm and 2am.

Between 2am and 6am the body enters a phase of psychic, mental and emotional repair. This is when we process all the information of the day. The idea of sleeping on something before making a decision

Power naps

Power naps are a short-term way of boosting the sleep you get. However, less than 60 minutes is best or you may disrupt your ability to sleep at night. Your brain dips into a different brainwave pattern when you nap, so it may take time to become alert again. Try going out in the daylight after a nap to reduce the feeling of jet lag!

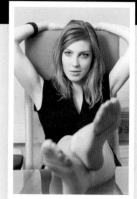

'Caffeine, diet, blood-sugar regulation, light, TVs, computers and mental and physical activity all affect our quality of sleep. Another factor is how dark our sleep environment is'

is very practical as you will process the information during the night.

Missing out on sleep between these hours has a detrimental effect. If you regularly go to sleep at 11pm that means you're missing out on a quarter of your physical repair time every single night. Add that up over the course of a whole year – or even a lifetime – and you can see how easy it is to rack up an enormous sleep debt! However, even if you sleep in until 7am you cannot make up that lost physical repair time, and the same applies to the other end of the night; getting up before 6am has the same effect on your psychic, mental and emotional repair.

If you find you don't feel tired enough to go to sleep by 10pm, this will largely be down to over-stimulation. By leaving the lights, computer and TV on late into the evening, we keep our brains active and inhibit the body's natural wind-down process, which is when we produce the hormones that make us feel sleepy. It takes a good couple of hours to reduce the effects of electric light stimulation so a period of preparation to sleep should occur from about 8pm.

However, if you immediately try to change the time you go to bed you are more likely to have problems sleeping. Instead, try gradually bringing your bedtime forwards by 15 minutes each week until you have achieved the target time.

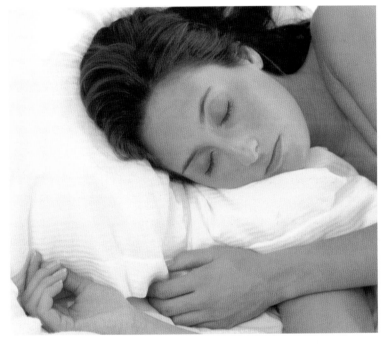

153

What factors affect the quality of our sleep?
Caffeinated drinks, diet, blood-sugar regulation, light, TVs, computers and mental and physical activity all affect our quality of sleep. Another important factor is how dark our sleep environment is. Any small chinks of light through curtains can register on the skin and stimulate the pineal gland to reduce its production of sleep hormones, so make your bedroom as dark as possible.

The effects on health
CHEK Practitioner and Holistic Lifestyle Coach Christine Bickley works with clients with various health issues and believes that sleep has a very important role when it comes to our health. She recommends that you try to get a minimum of eight hours' sleep a night during the summer and more in the winter, if possible. Make sure it's the best quality sleep possible and enjoy the benefits of improved health and vitality!

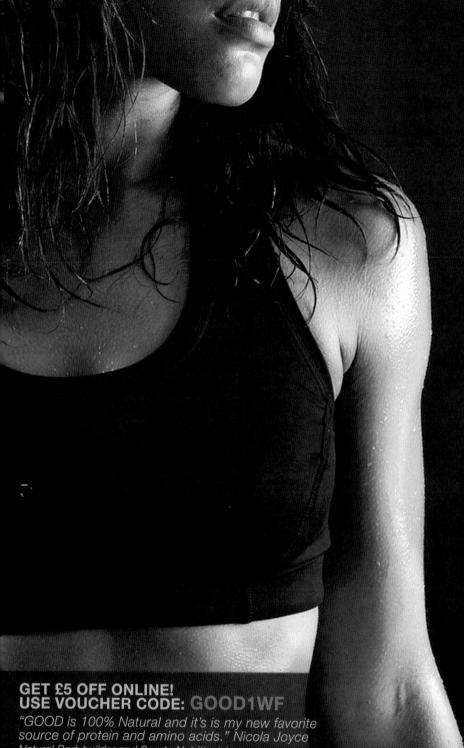
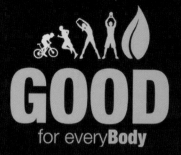
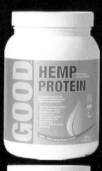

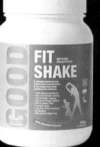

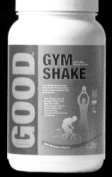

Nutrition

★ Food choices
★ Fat-burning foods
★ 8-week menu plan
★ Truth about fats

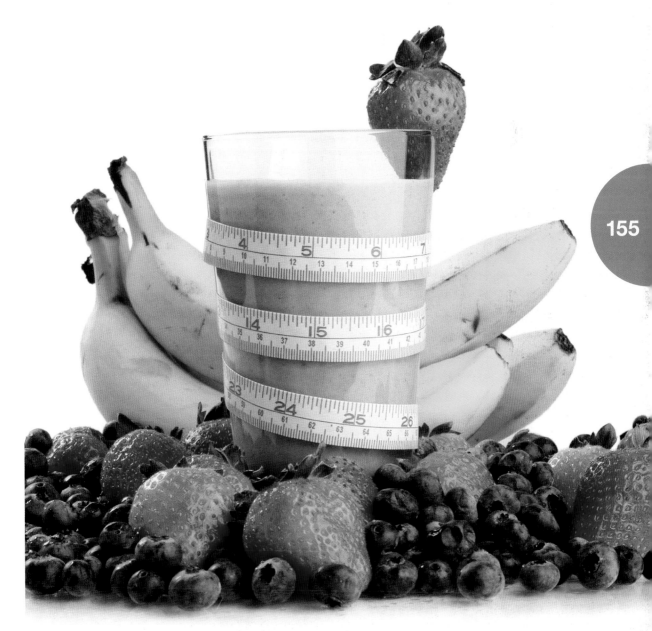

155

Body-boosting foods
Fuel your workout

Nutrition plays a vital role in improving your fitness, so ensure you're eating the right foods to complement your exercise routine

If you regularly work out, getting the right balance of carbs, protein, fats, vitamins and water is vital. We reveal the best foods to eat before and after exercise.

Energy for exercise
Carbohydrates (glucose) are the quickest and easiest form of energy for your body. They are either broken down into gylcogen (for instant energy) or glucagon (stored energy). Glycogen can only be stored for 24 hours so it is important that you load your body with complex/'good' carbs (like brown rice and wholegrains) at every meal, and in particular before endurance events like a long run or cycle, when you will be really pushing your body. It is also important not to load your body with refined sugar (e.g. white rice and pasta), as your body has no need for sugar when it's pushed to the limit. It will also burn off too quickly and leave you feeling more tired.

If you are going for a high-intensity gym session, make sure you have eaten an energy-filled snack (30-60 minutes) or meal (at least two hours) before your workout. This could be a low-GI option like wholegrain cereal with milk or, for a faster-releasing option, try three fig rolls or have a sports drink as they are specially formulated to provide the right balance.

Fat is also a necessary fuel, as it is the most energy-dense nutrient and provides many of the body's tissues and organs, including the heart, with most of their energy. Good examples include oily fish, olive oil, nuts, seeds and some meat and dairy.

The importance of water
During your workout it is important to stay hydrated – not just to replace the loss through sweating, but also to maintain a healthy balance of electrolytes so that your body performs at its optimum. Good hydration reduces the risk of

Refuelling snacks (eat within two hours post-exercise)

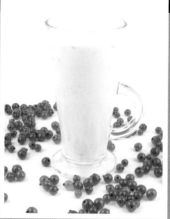

- One or two cartons of yogurt with berries and almonds
- A homemade milkshake
- A hot milky drink (hot chocolate or tea) with rye bread toast
- A tuna or cottage cheese sandwich on brown bread
- A handful of dried fruits and nuts
- A few rice cakes or oatcakes topped with peanut butter or houmous
- A bowl of porridge made with milk and honey
- A jacket potato with tuna or cottage cheese
- A smoothie (crushed fresh fruit whizzed in a blender)
- A couple of pieces of fresh fruit with a glass of milk
- A small salad with a sliced boiled egg
- Vegetable and bean soup
- An omelette with whatever you fancy

'The quicker you can get carbohydrate, protein and fluid into your body after your workout, the quicker your body will recover'

muscle damage, supports the immune system, aids recovery and ensures you get the most from your workout.

Food for recovery
It is just as important to refuel after a workout, as your glycogen stores are depleted and workouts can actually break down your muscle tissue. So, after exercise, you need to rebuild your fuel stores and provide your body with the right nutrients to repair damaged muscle fibres. Eat the wrong foods and you'll feel sluggish and tired for the rest of the day. Eat the right foods and you'll have more energy, feel stronger and recover faster.

When it comes to post-workout refuelling there is some debate about whether you should eat immediately after exercise, but this is more from a weight-management perspective. From a training perspective you should make use of what is known as 'the golden hour' after exercise and get some carbs back into your body as soon as possible. The quicker you can get carbohydrates, protein and fluid into your body after your workout, the quicker your body will recover from the stresses and strains you've put it through. The golden hour is the time when the muscles absorb the most nutrients and when the enzymes responsible for making them are most active, which leaves you just a few hours to reload your muscle glycogen. In fact, carbohydrate is converted into glycogen some one-and-a-half times faster than

Important nutrients to get in your diet

- Vitamin C is a powerful antioxidant and is required for tissue repair and helps boost the immune system.
- Potassium is needed for nerve and muscle function.
- Calcium is good for bone health and muscle function.
- B vitamins are important as they are required for the conversion of food into energy. B3, B6 and B12 are especially important in the storage of glycogen.
- Magnesium is essential for energy production. It is easily lost through sweating and low levels can lead to muscle fatigue.
- Omega-3 is especially important for runners. It's anti-inflammatory and therefore aids muscle repair between workouts.

157

normal straight after exercise. If you work out daily, speedy recovery is crucial, so have a carbohydrate-rich drink or snack as soon as possible after your workout, ideally within 30 minutes. Bananas, cereal bars, rice cakes or brown bread are perfect foods to eat following a workout.

Protein is also important for recovery, particularly when it comes to weight-training, as it helps muscles to repair and grow. Milk has been

shown to be effective after a workout, as well as lean white meats, fish, soya, beans and pulses. Whatever you decide to eat post-workout, these foods will provide you with sufficient levels of protein to help your muscles after a weight-bearing session.

Getting your nutritional balance right is essential for improving your stamina, speed, performance and recovery, so don't underestimate its importance.

Simple changes
Fat-burning food

Eating the right foods will really help your weight-loss efforts. Here are the key ingredients to add to your plate.

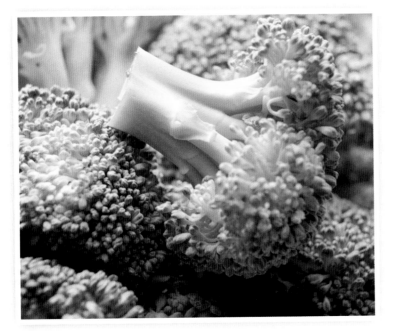

State University in America, soup is an appetite suppressant because it's made up of a hunger-satisfying combination of liquids and solids.

Broccoli boost
When you're trying to lose weight and shape up, non-starchy vegetables, such as broccoli, are one of the few foods that can be eaten in pretty much unlimited quantities. Broccoli contains cancer-fighting glucosinolates, as well as folate and vitamin C.

Brilliant barley
This milky-white grain has a rich, nut-like flavour and an appealing, chewy consistency. It's rich in soluble fibre, which helps to lower cholesterol levels and also controls hunger by slowing the rate at which sugar enters the bloodstream. Use it as an addition to soups and stews to bulk them up without adding excess calories.

Chew it over
Researchers have estimated that chewing sugar-free gum all day can increase your energy expenditure enough to burn off around 10 pounds a year. More to the point, while you're chewing gum, you can't eat anything else!

Nutty solution
Slimmers who eat a handful of almonds a day lose more weight than those who don't, according to

There's no quick fix for losing weight, but certain foods *can* help stabilise your blood sugar levels and keep you full.

An apple a day
This is a healthy snack, with a high water content and both kinds of weight-busting fibre – the soluble kind, which helps prevent blood sugar peaks that lead to cravings, and insoluble fibre, which helps fill you up.

Excellent eggs
Eggs are a great source of protein, and eating a high-protein diet is one of the key ways to stay full. In fact, a study in the *Journal Of The American College of Nutrition* found that when people ate two eggs for breakfast, they took in around 400 fewer calories over the next 24 hours than when they ate bagels.

Super soup
According to a study at Penn

'Opt for low-GI carbs, such as wholegrains, oats, whole fruit, yoghurt and beans'

American researchers. It's thought that the fat calories in almonds may not be completely absorbed. Nuts also contain fibre and protein, which makes them a satisfying snack that's great for your gym bag.

Good old grapefruit
In a study carried out by scientists at the Nutrition and Metabolic Research Centre at Scripps Clinic in San Diego, the simple act of adding grapefruit three times a day to the diets of obese people helped them to lose, on average, three-and-a-half pounds in 12 weeks, without making any other diet or activity changes.

Drink up!
Researchers in Germany found that subjects increased their metabolic rates (the rate at which calories are burned) by 30 per cent after drinking around 500ml of water. Drinking an extra one-and-a-half litres of water every day over the course of a year could mean a weight loss of approximately five pounds.

Go low
Low-fat dairy foods appear to slow down the process of making fat and increase fat burning, especially around the stomach. A study at the University of Tennessee found that dieters eating three servings of yogurt daily lost twice as much weight as their non-dairy eating counterparts.

Perfect porridge
Porridge is one of the best choices if you're trying to lose weight, as it's ranked as the most satiating breakfast food. Porridge slowly releases sugar into the system and helps you to stay fuller for longer.

Filling fish
Surprisingly, fish beats porridge in the satiety department. The Satiety Index ranks steamed white fish such as halibut or cod as the most filling food out of 38 common foods! Also, a study from Karolinska Institutet in Sweden found that people ate 11 per cent less at dinner after lunching on fish rather than beef.

Salad plate
Start your meal with a big plate of salad and you'll eat less overall. In a study, researchers at Penn State University found that women who ate a salad starter before a pasta lunch ate fewer calories over the course of the whole meal. Just make sure there are no calorific extras on top, like croutons or creamy dressing.

Keep it green
Substances called catechins in green tea appear to raise the metabolic rate slightly. By swapping five or six cups of standard tea for the same amount of green tea every day you'll burn up to an estimated 80 calories more per day.

159

Control cravings and beat hunger

- Eat breakfast to balance blood sugar for the day.
- Opt for low-GI carbs, such as wholegrains, oats, whole fruit (not juiced), yoghurt and beans. The body takes longer to digest low-GI carbs, and they also raise blood sugar levels much more slowly.
- Eat two decent servings of protein (meat, fish, eggs, tofu) a day. High-protein foods, as part of a mixed meal, help to slow the release of sugar into the bloodstream.
- Eat smaller portions more often to balance blood sugar.
- Include half a teaspoon of powdered cinnamon in your diet. The spice helps to maintain normal blood-sugar levels.

Get diet savvy
Eat smart to fight fat

The secret to shrinking your waistline can be added to your diet!
Include these five nutrients to reap the benefits

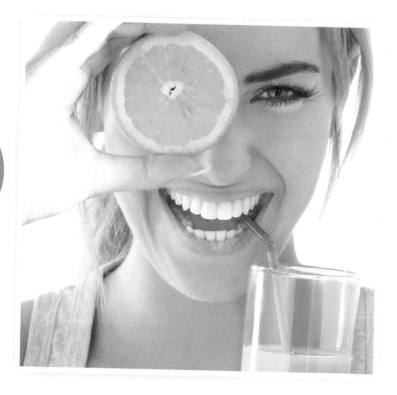

We all know that the first rule of losing weight is eating less and exercising more. But it's not just how much you eat, but *what* you eat that counts. You now know the type of foods that will help you stay fuller, longer, but there's also a whole host of nutrients that will actually accelerate your weight loss. 'The real key to any sort of sustainable

weight-loss programme is to focus on nutrient-dense foods rather than the low-calorie variety,' explains Stephanie Ridley, nutritional therapist at Nourish to Flourish (www.nourishtoflourish. com). 'You don't need to starve yourself to lose weight!' Here are the top five nutrients you should be scoffing to put your weight loss in the fast lane.

Omega-3 fatty acids

Omega-3 has many benefits, but did you know it could help you to lose weight? 'Omega-3 fatty acids support weight loss by increasing the enzymes involved in burning body fat,' says Stephanie. 'They are "essential": the body can't manufacture them, so they have to come from your diet.' The best way to utilise omega-3's fat-burning potential is to eat it. 'There are many omega-3 supplements on the market, but they vary in quality,' explains Stephanie. To boost your omega-3 intake, include plenty of oily fish, walnuts, linseed oil and eggs in your diet. **Try: Vitabiotics Ultra Omega-3 Fish Oil, £13.25 for 250ml, www.vitabiotics.com Top tip: Don't take omega-3 supplements if you're on anticoagulant medication, such as warfarin.**

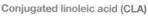

Conjugated linoleic acid (CLA)

This super nutrient is a naturally occurring fatty acid which may help to blitz the pounds. Numerous studies have shown that CLA helps the body to burn fat and build lean muscle tissue by reducing the uptake of fat into fat cells and boosting the breakdown of stored body fat. Decent levels are found in dairy products, safflower oil and beef, but taking a daily

'You don't need to starve
yourself to lose weight!'

dose of 3,200mg in supplement form has been shown to help reduce body fat safely in eight to 12 weeks.
Try: Reflex CLA, £13.76, www.reflex-nutrition.com
Top tip: **Take with main meals for best results.**

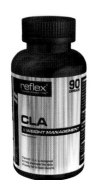

Chromium
'Chromium is needed to carry sugar from the blood into your body's cells, where it can then be burned for energy,' says Stephanie. 'But, if this process doesn't happen efficiently, any sugar remaining in the blood may be converted into body fat, which can lead to weight gain.'
We all make an effort to cut out some of the unnecessary sugar from our diets, but how many of us are guilty of having an extra biscuit with our tea, or opting for white carbs over brown?
'If you often choose sugary or refined carbs over wholegrain versions, you increase your need for chromium,' says Stephanie. If this sounds familiar, try to cut back on the refined carbs you eat, switching them for low-GI options like sweet potato, and top up with foods rich in chromium.

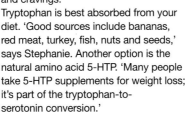

'It's found in wholegrains, romaine lettuce, raw onions and tomatoes, and in most good-quality multivitamin supplements,' Stephanie adds.
Try: BioCare NutriSorb Chromium, £16.50, www.biocare.co.uk
Top tip: **Insulin-dependent diabetics should consult their doctor before taking chromium as their insulin may need adjusting.**

Tryptophan
'Tryptophan is an amino acid that the body converts to serotonin, needed for normal appetite control,' says Stephanie. 'Low levels of serotonin are thought to increase appetite and cravings.'
Tryptophan is best absorbed from your diet. 'Good sources include bananas, red meat, turkey, fish, nuts and seeds,' says Stephanie. Another option is the natural amino acid 5-HTP. 'Many people take 5-HTP supplements for weight loss; it's part of the tryptophan-to-serotonin conversion.'
Try: Solgar 5-HTP, £10.17, www.revital.com
Top tip: **People on antidepressants should consult their doctor before taking 5-HTP supplements.**

Iodine
The final fat burner is an important weapon in the fight against weight gain. 'Iodine is a vital component of the thyroid gland's function, which regulates your metabolism,' says Stephanie.
'If your metabolism is low, you're likely to struggle with weight.'
The easiest way to add iodine to your diet is to stock up on seafood. 'It's found in white fish, shellfish and seaweed,' notes Stephanie. Or, try eggs, yoghurt and potatoes for an iodine-rich feast.
Try: Avogel kelp tablets, £6.10, www.avogel.co.uk
Top tip: **As with all supplements, don't start taking iodine supplements without consulting a doctor or health professional first.**

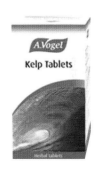

161

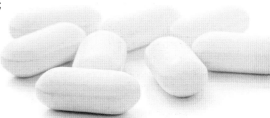

Lose a stone in eight weeks. Yes, it's true, it can be done. You can lose a stone without resorting to a crazy fad diet or killing yourself in the gym. Simply follow our nutritionally balanced eight-week plan...

Week 1

Each day's calorific intake is based on small portions. Lower calorie intake allows for two whey protein drinks a day to be taken in conjunction with the diet if in training or to ensure a feeling of fullness and to avoid snacking

	Monday	Tuesday	Wednesday
Breakfast	• 2 grilled tomatoes • 1 poached/coddled egg • 2 slices rye bread • 150ml glass of fresh orange juice	• 140g porridge oats made with water, topped with a handful of chopped walnuts • 150ml glass of fresh orange juice	• Smoothie made with 250ml soya milk, 1 pear, 1 peach, 1 banana, 2 apricots and fresh mint, topped with 1tbsp ground sunflower seeds • 1 slice wholemeal toast
Mid-morning snacks	• Small bunch of grapes • 1 apple	• 100g reduced-fat cottage cheese with 2 celery sticks, 1 raw courgette and 1 carrot stick	• Handful of raspberries • 150g low-fat yogurt
Lunch	• Grilled 100g minute steak with 2 sliced tomatoes and 4 lettuce leaves • 1 large wholewheat pitta bread	• 100g baked potato with small tin of tuna and 2tbsps of sweetcorn	• 100g grilled chicken breast with 25g sliced avocado, 1 sliced tomato, 20g watercress and lemon juice • 2 slices rye bread
Mid-afternoon snacks	• 100g low-fat fruit yogurt • 100g strawberries	• 200g yogurt drink • 1 apricot • Handful of raspberries	• 2 raw carrots • 2 celery sticks • Handful of cucumber sticks
Dinner	• 100g steamed lemon sole • 2 small steamed broccoli spears • 1 grated raw medium courgette • 200g baked potato	• Beef and lentil curry: 125g oven-cooked beef with 25g lentils, 50g steamed okra and 150g curry sauce • 75g brown rice	• Spaghetti Bolognese: 100g mince and 150g Bolognese sauce • 60g spaghetti
Total daily intake	cals 1,497 protein 89g fat 35g carbs 220g fibre 20g	cals 1,628 protein 108g fat 48g carbs 204g fibre 16g	cals 1,493 protein 96g fat 57g carbs 158g fibre 23g

162

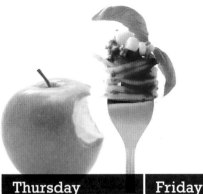

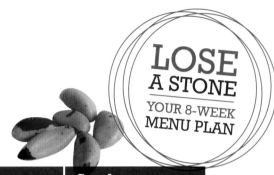

LOSE
A STONE
YOUR 8-WEEK
MENU PLAN

Thursday	Friday	Saturday	Sunday
• 40g All Bran cereal with 100ml soya milk • 100g low-fat plain yogurt with 100g fresh strawberries and 3 chopped Brazil nuts • 150ml glass of fresh grapefruit juice	• 40g Bran flakes with 100ml skimmed milk • 1 boiled egg • 150ml glass of fresh orange juice	• 4tbsps of soya or bio yogurt with a handful of mixed chopped nuts and sunflower seeds • 1 slice wholemeal toast • 150ml glass of fresh grapefruit juice	• Smoothie made with 250ml soya milk, 1tbsp of ground sunflower seeds, ½ mango, 100g raspberries, 4 rings fresh pineapple, 1 orange and 1 chopped grapefruit
• 2 oatcakes • 6 almonds	• 1 apple • 2 oatcakes • Vegetable juice: 2 beetroots, 30g cucumber, ginger and 3 celery sticks	• 1 apple • Handful of Brazil nuts	• 150g low-fat fruit yogurt with a handful of mixed nuts
• 200g baked potato with small tin of tuna and 2tbsps of sweetcorn	• Mixed bean salad: 1tbsp of each of the following: azuki, soya, butter and mung beans, fresh olives, fresh mint, olive oil and chopped tomato, served with 100g grilled chicken breast	• 200g baked potato with 100g reduced sugar and salt baked beans	• Greek salad: 50g diced feta cheese, 20g pitted black olives, 20g cucumber, 1 tomato, 40g onion, oregano and olive oil • 2 small wholemeal pitta breads
• 6 dried apricots	• Small bunch of grapes	• 25g tzatziki with vegetable sticks: 1 carrot, 30g cucumber, 1 celery stick and ½ red pepper	• Vegetable juice: 2 celery sticks, 30g cucumber, 2 carrots and handful of mint
• 120g grilled haddock fillet • Handful of pre-cooked prawns, 2 sprigs of parsley, 20g watercress, 120g tomatoes, 70g beetroot, 75g red onion and French dressing • 150g sweet potato mash	• 100g grilled fillet steak • 100g French beans • 50g mange tout • 130g sweet baked potato	• Lamb steak stir-fry: 100g lamb steak, 20g bean sprouts, 1 broccoli spear, 20g cabbage, 20g green pepper, 30g sweetcorn, 20g mange tout, 20g chestnuts and 10g soy sauce	• 120g grilled halibut steak drizzled with lime juice • 60g grated raw courgette • 80g steamed chicory • 100g runner beans
cals 1,432 protein 91g fat 37g carbs 196g fibre 26g	cals 1,465 protein 101g fat 44g carbs 176g fibre 33g	cals 1,368 protein 65g fat 61g carbs 149g fibre 22g	cals 1,444 protein 73g fat 51g carbs 185g fibre 24g

163

Week 2

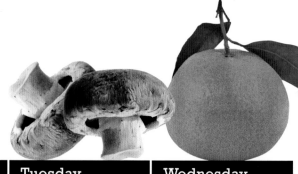

	Monday	Tuesday	Wednesday
Breakfast	• 2 grilled tomatoes • 3 large mushrooms • 1 poached/coddled egg • 1 slice wholemeal toast • 150ml glass of fresh orange juice	• 140g porridge oats made with water • Vegetable juice: 3 celery sticks, 2 carrots, 2 beetroots, 1 apple, pinch of ginger and 2 apricots	• 6 stewed prunes • 50g Bran Flakes with 100ml skimmed milk
Mid-morning snacks	• 2 small tangerines • 30g houmous with 1 carrot and 50g green pepper sticks	• 150g low-fat plain yogurt with 100g blackberries, 10g ground sesame seeds and 10g sunflower seeds	• 150g low-fat yogurt • Handful of Brazil nuts
Lunch	• 100g reduced sugar and salt baked beans • 2 slices seeded granary toast • 150g low-fat plain yogurt with 100g blackberries • 1 apricot	• Small tin of anchovy fillets, 4 lettuce leaves, 1 sliced tomato, 60g red onion, 20g cucumber and French dressing • 1 wholemeal roll	• 120g grilled chicken breast with 60g azuki beans, 30g alfalfa sprouts and 1 chopped tomato • 1 wholemeal roll
Mid-afternoon snacks	• 2 oatcakes • 6 Brazil nuts	• 150g low-fat fruit yogurt • Handful of almonds	• 100g strawberries • 1 apple
Dinner	• 100g steamed lemon sole • 3 steamed broccoli spears • 125g spinach • 1 raw grated medium courgette • 200g baked potato	• Beef stir-fry: 125g lean beef, 60g red pepper and 60g green pepper, 9ml sesame oil, 5ml soy sauce, 3 garlic cloves and 100g broccoli spears	• 120g grilled salmon steak • 90g steamed spinach • 90g runner beans • 175g minted new potatoes
Total daily intake	**cals** 1,454 **protein** 80g **fat** 42g **carbs** 201g **fibre** 32g	**cals** 1,327 **protein** 80g **fat** 52g **carbs** 141g **fibre** 27g	**cals** 1,511 **protein** 85g **fat** 57g **carbs** 174g **fibre** 28g

164

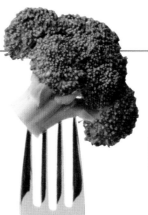

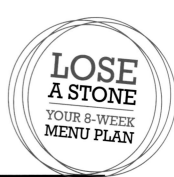

LOSE
A STONE
YOUR 8-WEEK
MENU PLAN

Thursday	Friday	Saturday	Sunday
• Omelette made with 2 egg whites and 3 chopped asparagus stems • 2 slices wholemeal toast • 150ml glass of fresh orange juice	• 2 grilled tomatoes • 3 large mushrooms • 2 slices rye bread • 150ml glass of fresh grapefruit juice	• 140g porridge oats made with water • Vegetable juice: 2 celery sticks, 2 carrots, 2 beetroots, pinch of ginger and 30g cucumber	• 1 slice wholemeal toast and yeast spread • 150g low-fat plain yogurt with 100g strawberries and 3 chopped Brazil nuts • 150ml glass of fresh grapefruit juice
• Handful of mixed nuts • 150g low-fat fruit yogurt	• 150g soya yogurt with 25g Brazil nuts and 100g strawberries	• 150g low-fat fruit yogurt with handful of sesame seeds • 1 apple	• Smoothie made with 250ml soya milk, 1 banana, 10g honey, 1 kiwi fruit and 100g raspberries
• Small tin of tuna, 30g azuki beans and 30g black-eyed beans with 7g lemon juice and 20g olives	• 200g baked potato with 100g sweetcorn and 50g low-fat cottage cheese	• 45g smoked salmon, lemon juice and black pepper • 2 slices wholemeal bread	• 300g tomato soup topped with watercress • 1 wholegrain roll • 1 orange • 1 pear • 3 figs
• 2 satsumas • 2 apricots	• 1 peach • 1 orange	• 2 tangerines • 1 pear	• 20g tzatziki with 1 carrot stick and 1 celery stick • Handful of walnuts
• Diced lamb curry: 125g oven-cooked lamb, 25g dhal and 150g curry sauce • 50g brown rice	• 200g steamed trout with 10g almonds • 100g broccoli • 50g mange tout • 160g new potatoes	• Lamb biryani: 300g lamb, 25g lentils, 25g okra and 4 slices of mango	• 120g grilled halibut steak with dill • 125g creamed spinach • 150g baked sweet potato
cals 1,594 protein 102g fat 51g carbs 194g fibre 22g	cals 1,416 protein 79g fat 40g carbs 196g fibre 23g	cals 1,696 protein 62g fat 65g carbs 229g fibre 25g	cals 1,454 protein 66g fat 45g carbs 207g fibre 27g

165

Week 3

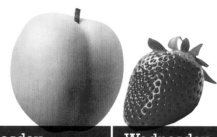

	Monday	Tuesday	Wednesday
Breakfast	• 2 scrambled eggs • 2 grilled tomatoes • 2 slices wholemeal toast • 150ml glass of fresh orange juice	• 140g porridge oats made with water topped with 10g sunflower seeds and 20g mixed nuts • 1 slice rye bread with 4 grilled mushrooms	• Smoothie made with 250ml soya milk, 1 pear, 1 peach, 2 apricots and topped with 1tbsp ground sunflower/flaxseeds • 1 slice granary toast
Mid-morning snacks	• 150g low-fat yogurt • 1 apple • 1 pear • 1 satsuma	• 150g low-fat yogurt • Small bunch of grapes • 1 apple	• 2 nectarines • Handful of mixed nuts
Lunch	• 50g noodles with 75g grilled tiger prawns, parsley, lemon juice and 1 chopped spring onion	• 25g pre-cooked prawns and lemon juice with 125g chopped avocado and 1 tomato • 2 slices granary bread	• 295g bowl of watercress soup topped with 20g watercress • 1 wholemeal roll
Mid-afternoon snacks	• 25g houmous with vegetable sticks: 1 carrot, 75g red pepper and 2 celery sticks	• 45g taramasalata with 2 inches cucumber chopped into sticks • Handful of blackberries • 1 orange	• Handful of dried apricots
Dinner	• Chicken curry with coriander: 125g chicken and 15g curry sauce • 50g brown rice	• 125g grilled fillet steak with 130g tomato sauce • 50g wholemeal pasta	• 125g grilled gammon steak with 150g fresh grapefruit segments • 100g runner beans • 200g baked potato
Total daily intake	**cals** 1,619 **protein** 90g **fat** 59g **carbs** 194g **fibre** 18g	**cals** 1,572 **protein** 77g **fat** 67g **carbs** 175g **fibre** 23g	**cals** 1,448 **protein** 64g **fat** 48g **carbs** 200g **fibre** 27g

166

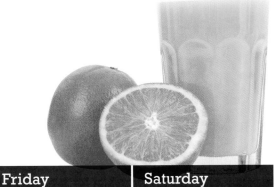
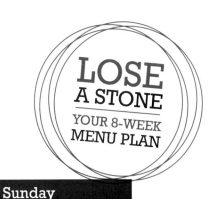

LOSE A STONE
YOUR 8-WEEK
MENU PLAN

Thursday	Friday	Saturday	Sunday
• 40g sugar-free muesli with 100ml skimmed milk • 1 poached/coddled egg • 1 slice brown bread • 150ml glass of fresh orange juice	• 30g Bran Flakes with 100ml skimmed milk, topped with handful of blackberries • 2 apricots • 150ml glass of fresh grapefruit juice	• 1 grilled kipper topped with a poached egg and drizzled with lemon juice and parsley • 1 slice granary bread	• Omelette made with 2 egg whites, 10g cheese, 50g red pepper, 50g green pepper and 4 mushrooms • 2 slices rye bread • 150ml glass of fresh orange juice
• 150g soya yogurt and 100g strawberries/ blueberries/ cherries	• 1 orange • 50g cottage cheese with 1 carrot and 30g cucumber sticks	• 2 satsumas • Handful of Brazil nuts • 150ml glass of fresh orange juice	• Fruit juice: 300g watermelon, pinch of ginger, 1 apple and 1 mango • Handful of walnuts
• 125g grilled minute steak with 1 chopped apple, 1 celery stick, handful of alfalfa sprouts and 1 beetroot • 2 small pitta breads	• 125g smoked mackerel with fresh lemon juice 20g watercress, 50g beetroot and 4 slices red onion • 1 wholemeal roll	• 200g baked potato with 60g reduced sugar and salt baked beans	• 100g reduced sugar and salt baked beans • 2 slices granary toast
• Vegetable juice: 150g watermelon, 2 tomatoes, 30g cucumber and handful of mint	• Smoothie made with 250ml soya milk, 1tbsp flaxseed/ sunflower seeds, 1 mango and 100g raspberries	• 150g Greek yogurt with 100g strawberries	• 1 pear • 1 orange • 50g cottage cheese with 1 carrot and 40g celery sticks
• 100g grilled sardines with parsley • 4 lettuce leaves, ½ red onion, 50g red peppers, 20g watercress with 7g olive oil and lemon juice dressing • 120g new potatoes	• Chicken curry: 125g oven-cooked chicken, 125g spinach, 25g chickpeas and 150g curry sauce • 50g brown rice	• Chilli con carne: 50g pan-fried mince, 220g chilli con carne sauce and 10g Parmesan cheese • 50g brown rice	• 150g grilled fillet haddock with parsley • 125g creamed spinach • 100g peas • 160g minted new potatoes
cals 1,664 protein 103g **fat** 52g **carbs** 207g **fibre** 17g	**cals 1,708 protein** 98g **fat** 69g **carbs** 185g **fibre** 27g	**cals 1,669 protein** 96g **fat** 65g **carbs** 186g **fibre** 20g	**cals 1,483 protein** 81g **fat** 34g **carbs** 227g **fibre** 36g

167

Week 4

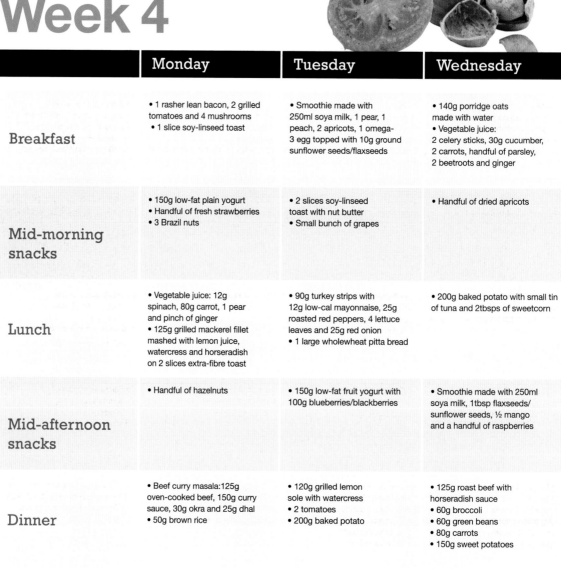

	Monday	Tuesday	Wednesday
Breakfast	• 1 rasher lean bacon, 2 grilled tomatoes and 4 mushrooms • 1 slice soy-linseed toast	• Smoothie made with 250ml soya milk, 1 pear, 1 peach, 2 apricots, 1 omega-3 egg topped with 10g ground sunflower seeds/flaxseeds	• 140g porridge oats made with water • Vegetable juice: 2 celery sticks, 30g cucumber, 2 carrots, handful of parsley, 2 beetroots and ginger
Mid-morning snacks	• 150g low-fat plain yogurt • Handful of fresh strawberries • 3 Brazil nuts	• 2 slices soy-linseed toast with nut butter • Small bunch of grapes	• Handful of dried apricots
Lunch	• Vegetable juice: 12g spinach, 80g carrot, 1 pear and pinch of ginger • 125g grilled mackerel fillet mashed with lemon juice, watercress and horseradish on 2 slices extra-fibre toast	• 90g turkey strips with 12g low-cal mayonnaise, 25g roasted red peppers, 4 lettuce leaves and 25g red onion • 1 large wholewheat pitta bread	• 200g baked potato with small tin of tuna and 2tbsps of sweetcorn
Mid-afternoon snacks	• Handful of hazelnuts	• 150g low-fat fruit yogurt with 100g blueberries/blackberries	• Smoothie made with 250ml soya milk, 1tbsp flaxseeds/ sunflower seeds, ½ mango and a handful of raspberries
Dinner	• Beef curry masala:125g oven-cooked beef, 150g curry sauce, 30g okra and 25g dhal • 50g brown rice	• 120g grilled lemon sole with watercress • 2 tomatoes • 200g baked potato	• 125g roast beef with horseradish sauce • 60g broccoli • 60g green beans • 80g carrots • 150g sweet potatoes
Total daily intake	cals 1,734 **protein** 104g **fat** 78g **carbs** 163g **fibre** 18g	cals 1,443 **protein** 95g **fat** 31g **carbs** 208g **fibre** 20g	cals 1,511 **protein** 97g **fat** 39g **carbs** 204g **fibre** 32g

168

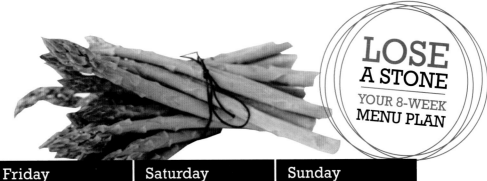

LOSE
A STONE
YOUR 8-WEEK
MENU PLAN

Thursday	Friday	Saturday	Sunday
• Omelette made with 1 egg yolk, 4 egg whites and 4 mushrooms • 1 slice wholemeal toast • 150ml glass of fresh orange juice	• 1 grapefruit cut into segments • 30g muesli with 100ml skimmed milk • 1 slice granary toast • 150ml glass of fresh orange juice	• Smoothie made with 250ml soya milk, 1 pear, 1 peach and 2 apricots • 1 boiled egg • 2 slices wholemeal toast	• Omelette made with 2 egg whites and 3 chopped asparagus stems and tips • 2 slices wholemeal toast • 150ml glass of fresh orange juice
• 150g low-fat yogurt with handful of blueberries or blackberries	• 1 apple • 2 tangerines	• 150g low-fat yogurt with a handful of raspberries • 1 orange	• 35g reduced-fat cottage cheese with 1 carrot and 80g celery sticks
• 2 slices roast chicken, 5g cress and 5 slices avocado • 1 wholemeal pitta bread • 1 orange	• 315g watercress soup with 1 granary roll • 1 nectarine • 1 pear	• 125g kedgeree with watercress	• 200g baked potato with small tin of tuna • 10g azuki beans, 10g black-eyed beans, 7g lemon juice and 20g olives
• 25g tzatziki with 2 carrot sticks and 1 celery stick • Handful of hazelnuts	• 25g houmous with 60g raw courgette and 40g celery sticks • 1 orange	• Handful of raspberries and blackcurrants	• 150g plain yogurt • 2 oatcakes • 1 orange • 1 pear
• 200g grilled trout with 10g almonds and lemon juice • 4 lettuce leaves, 50g green peppers, 50g red onion, 20g watercress, 2 tomatoes and French dressing	• Chicken and red pepper casserole: 125g chicken and 50g red peppers • 25g creamed spinach • 100g runner beans • 200g baked potato	• Spaghetti Bolognese: 75g mince and 250g Bolognese sauce • 50g wholemeal spaghetti	• Diced lamb and chickpea curry: 100g diced lamb, 25g chick peas, 150g curry sauce and 25g dhal • 50g brown rice
cals 1,345 protein 82g fat 53g carbs 142g fibre 20g	**cals 1,408 protein 69g fat 20g carbs 253g fibre 33g**	**cals 1,461 protein 83g fat 64g carbs 148g fibre 21g**	**cals 1,796 protein 106g fat 46g carbs 254g fibre 25g**

169

Week 5

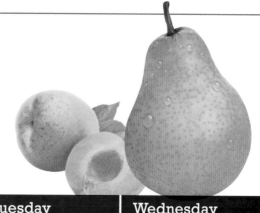

	Monday	Tuesday	Wednesday
Breakfast	• 1 poached egg • 2 grilled tomatoes • 2 slices wholemeal toast • 150ml glass of fresh orange juice	• 140g porridge oats with water • 2 slices wholemeal toast with nut butter • 150ml glass of fresh orange juice	• Smoothie made with 250ml soya milk, 1 pear, 1 peach, 2 apricots and topped with 10g ground sunflower seeds/flaxseeds • 1 slice wholemeal toast
Mid-morning snacks	• 150g low-fat yogurt with handful of almonds • Handful of strawberries	• Vegetable juice: 2 celery sticks, 2 carrots, 2 beetroots, 1 apple and pinch of ginger • 1 low-fat yogurt • Small bunch of grapes	• 2 nectarines • Handful of mixed nuts
Lunch	• 50g noodles with 100g crab, lemon juice and 12g chilli peppers • 1 wholemeal roll	• 30g pre-cooked prawns and 125g avocado with lemon juice • 2 slices granary bread	• 315g bowl of watercress soup • 1 wholemeal roll
Mid-afternoon snacks	• 25g tzatziki with 1 carrot and 1 celery stick	• 2 rye crispbreads with 25g cottage cheese • 1 orange • Handful of blackberries/blueberries	• 2 apricots • 2 oatcakes
Dinner	• Chicken and okra curry: 125g oven-cooked chicken, 50g okra and 150g curry sauce • 50g brown rice • 1 naan bread	• 125g grilled fillet steak with 130g tomato sauce • 50g wholewheat spaghetti	• 250g moussaka with 20g watercress, 1 tomato and 50g onion salad
Total daily intake	**cals** 1,750 **protein** 100g **fat** 59g **carbs** 217g **fibre** 19g	**cals** 1,574 **protein** 84g **fat** 47g **carbs** 215g **fibre** 31g	**cals** 1,465 **protein** 60g **fat** 71g **carbs** 156g **fibre** 22g

170

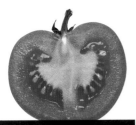

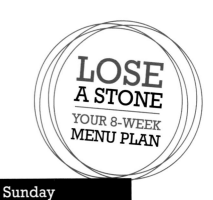

LOSE A STONE
YOUR 8-WEEK MENU PLAN

171

Thursday	Friday	Saturday	Sunday
• 2 scrambled eggs • 1 slice soy-linseed toast • 150ml glass of fresh grapefruit juice	• 100g fresh raspberries • 1 boiled egg • 2 wholemeal slices toast • 150ml glass of fresh grapefruit juice	• 120g grilled kipper, 2 tomatoes and 4 mushrooms drizzled with lemon juice	• 2 scrambled eggs • 2 wholemeal slices toast • 150ml glass of fresh orange juice
• 150g low-fat yogurt with handful of strawberries	• 1 orange • 1 pear	• 2 satsumas • Handful of Brazil nuts • 150ml glass of fresh orange juice	• Vegetable juice: 2 celery sticks, 2 carrots, 1 beetroot and pinch of ginger
• 125g grilled chicken, 1 chopped apple, 1 celery stick, 25g chickpeas, 10g alfalfa sprouts and 7g olive oil and lemon juice dressing	• 125g smoked mackerel with fresh lemon juice, 20g watercress and 30g cucumber • 2 slices rye bread	• 200g baked potato with 100g reduced sugar and salt baked beans	• 125g grilled minute steak and 20g watercress • 2 slices granary bread
• 25g houmous on 2 rye crispbreads • 1 orange • Handful of blackberries/ blueberries	• Smoothie made with 250ml soya milk, 1 mango and handful of raspberries	• 150g low-fat yogurt with a handful of strawberries	• 50g cottage cheese and 75g cucumber sticks
• 120g grilled plaice with lemon juice • 100g peas • 100g sweetcorn • 150g baked sweet potato	• Chicken curry: 150g oven-cooked chicken and 150g curry sauce • 50g brown rice	• 125g grilled fillet steak • 100g steamed broccoli • 100g runner beans • 200g baked sweet potato	• 150g haddock fillet • 2 tomatoes, 50g beetroot and 75g red onion with 7g lemon juice • 200g baked potato
cals 1,524 protein 90g fat 52g carbs 186g fibre 24g	cals 1,432 protein 87g fat 68g carbs 124g fibre 18g	cals 1,479 protein 93g fat 44g carbs 189g fibre 24g	cals 1,597 protein 110g fat 56g carbs 174g fibre 22g

Week 6

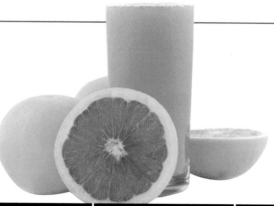

	Monday	Tuesday	Wednesday
Breakfast	• 2 slices wholemeal toast with 4 mushrooms • 150g low-fat plain yogurt with 100g fresh strawberries and 3 chopped Brazil nuts • 150ml glass of fresh grapefruit juice	• 6 stewed prunes • 30g Bran Flakes with 100ml skimmed milk • 150ml glass of fresh ruby red grapefruit juice	• 1 grapefruit cut into segments • 2 boiled eggs • 2 slices rye bread • 150ml glass of fresh orange juice
Mid-morning snacks	• Vegetable juice: 2 carrots, 2 tomatoes, 2 celery sticks and handful of parsley	• 150g low-fat yogurt with a handful of blackberries and sunflower seeds/flaxseeds	• Vegetable juice: 2 inches cucumber, pinch of ginger and 3 celery sticks • 2 oatcakes
Lunch	• 100g grilled turkey breast, 20g watercress, 25g soya beans, 5 slices of red peppers with 7g lemon juice and olive oil dressing • 2 rye crispbreads	• 125g smoked mackerel fillet with lemon juice • 2 slices wholemeal toast	• 45g poached/grilled salmon and 6 slices cucumber • 2 slices wholemeal bread
Mid-afternoon snacks	• Handful of mixed nuts	• 1 banana • 100g strawberries	• 1 pear • 1 orange • Handful of Brazil nuts
Dinner	• 155g steamed trout • Mixed salad: 50g green peppers, 3 slices red onion, 20g cucumber, 4 lettuce leaves and 35g beetroot • 200g baked potato	• 100g roast beef • 100g broccoli • 100g green beans • 25g soya beans • 2 small roasted sweet potatoes	• Chicken and spinach curry: 125g oven-cooked chicken, 125g spinach, 150g curry sauce and handful of chopped apricots • 50g brown rice
Total daily intake	**cals** 1,490 **protein** 106g **fat** 44g **carbs** 177g **fibre** 29g	**cals** 1,527 **protein** 88g **fat** 66g **carbs** 155g **fibre** 24g	**cals** 1,467 **protein** 78g **fat** 50g **carbs** 186g **fibre** 22g

172

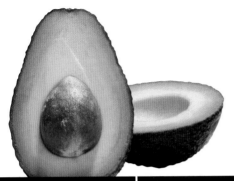

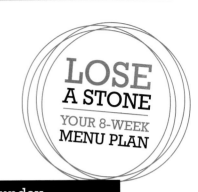

LOSE
A STONE
YOUR 8-WEEK
MENU PLAN

Thursday	Friday	Saturday	Sunday
• 1 poached egg • 2 grilled tomatoes • 4 mushrooms • 2 slices wholemeal toast • 150ml glass of fresh orange juice	• 40g sugar-free muesli with 100ml semi-skimmed milk, 1 banana and 1 kiwi fruit • 2 slices wholemeal toast with nut butter • 150ml glass of fresh orange juice	• 4tbsps of yogurt with strawberries • 2 scrambled eggs made with 135ml milk • 150ml glass of fresh grapefruit juice	• 2 grilled tomatoes • 1 poached/coddled egg • 2 slices rye bread • 150ml glass of fresh orange juice
• 150g low-fat yogurt with 10g sunflower seeds	• 150g low-fat fruit yogurt • 1 apricot	• Handful of dried apricots • 1 orange • 25g cottage cheese on 2 rye crispbreads	• 25g tzatziki with 2 carrot sticks
• 50g prawns and 1 sliced avocado with squeeze of lemon juice • 2 slices rye bread	• 125g grilled chicken breast with 1 tomato, 2 spring onions and 4 lettuce leaves • 1 large wholewheat pitta bread	• 100g reduced sugar and salt baked beans • 2 slices wholemeal toast	• 75g smoked mackerel fillet with squeeze of lemon juice and 20g watercress • 2 slices granary toast
• 100g raspberries • 25g tzatziki with 80g celery sticks and 40g carrot sticks	• 100g blackberries • 40g low-fat cottage cheese on 2 rye crispbreads	• Small bunch of grapes • 150ml glass of fresh orange juice	• Handful of strawberries • 150g fruit yogurt
• 125g flash-grilled chicken escalope with squeeze of lemon juice, 65g roasted aubergine, 50g courgette and 50g red peppers • 200g baked potato	• 125g grilled gammon steak with 125g fresh grapefruit segments • 100g broad beans • 100g runner beans • 150g baked sweet potato	• 175g salmon steak • 100g spinach • 100g runner beans • 160g new potatoes	• 125g grilled fillet steak • 100g broccoli • 100g green beans • 25g soya beans • 150g roasted sweet potatoes
cals 1,324 **protein** 80g **fat** 42g **carbs** 166g **fibre** 24g	**cals** 1,738 **protein** 99g **fat** 44g **carbs** 250g **fibre** 31g	**cals** 1,430 **protein** 87g **fat** 58g **carbs** 148g **fibre** 23g	**cals** 1,504 **protein** 94g **fat** 60g **carbs** 154g **fibre** 23g

173

Week 7

	Monday	Tuesday	Wednesday
Breakfast	• 140g porridge oats with water • Vegetable juice: 2 celery sticks, 125g spinach, parsley, 2 carrots and 1 beetroot	• 150g soya yogurt with handful of blackberries • 1 boiled or coddled egg • 2 slices soy-linseed bread • 150ml glass of fresh grapefruit juice	• 140g porridge oats with water • 2 slices wholemeal toast • Vegetable juice: 2 celery sticks, 125g spinach, 1 beetroot, 1 apple and pinch of ginger
Mid-morning snacks	• Smoothie made with 250ml soya milk, 10g ground flaxseed/ sunflower seeds, ½ mango and a handful of raspberries	• 25g houmous dip with 2 carrots • 1 apple • 1 pear	• 150g low-fat yogurt • Small bunch of grapes
Lunch	• 56g smoked salmon and 30g cucumber • 2 slices wholemeal bread	• 200g baked potato with small tin of tuna and 2tbsps of sweetcorn	• 125g grilled chicken, 1 small avocado and few sprigs of basil • 2 slices rye bread
Mid-afternoon snacks	• 2 apricots • 1 apple • 2 oatcakes	• 150g soya yogurt topped with handful of sunflower seeds • 2 satsumas	• 2 crispbreads with 25g cottage cheese • 200g slice of watermelon
Dinner	• Chicken lentil and spinach curry: 125g oven-cooked chicken, 25g lentils, 125g spinach, 150g curry sauce • 50g brown rice • 2 chapatis	• 125g grilled fillet steak • 100g steamed broccoli • 125g spinach • 100g runner beans • 150g creamed sweet potato mash	• 120g steamed lemon sole with lemon juice • 25g soya beans • 3 broccoli spears • 1 raw grated medium courgette • 200g new potatoes
Total daily intake	cals 1,572 protein 91g fat 39g carbs 226g fibre 22g	cals 1,757 protein 114g fat 50g carbs 227g fibre 33g	cals 1,407 protein 98g fat 40g carbs 174g fibre 29g

174

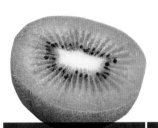
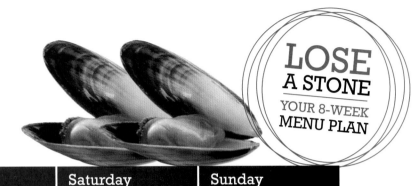

LOSE
A STONE
YOUR 8-WEEK
MENU PLAN

Thursday	Friday	Saturday	Sunday
• 2 grilled tomatoes • 1 poached/coddled egg • 1 slice soy-linseed bread • 150ml glass of fresh orange juice • 2 small tangerines	• Smoothie made with 150g low-fat yogurt, 1 pear, 1 peach and 1 apricot, topped with 10g ground sunflower seeds • 4 grilled mushrooms • 1 slice wholemeal toast	• Smoothie made with 150g low-fat yogurt, 1 pear, 1 peach and 2 apricots • 100g reduced sugar and salt beans • 2 slices wholemeal toast	• 1 kipper topped with a poached egg and slice of lemon • 1 slice wholemeal toast • 200g yogurt drink • 150ml glass of fresh orange juice
• Smoothie with 150g low-fat yogurt, handful of Brazil nuts, 100g strawberries and 1 peach	• 150g low-fat yogurt with 100g raspberries • 2 rye crispbreads with 30g mackerel	• 100g raspberries • Handful of hazelnuts	• 150g low-fat yogurt • 1 apple • 1 pear
• 200g baked potato with 100g reduced sugar and salt baked beans	• 40g pre-cooked prawns, 125g avocado, 20g watercress, 12g mayonnaise and squeeze of lemon juice • 2 slices wholemeal bread with low-fat spread	• 295g watercress soup topped with extra 20g watercress • 1 wholemeal roll	• 100g grilled minute steak with 20g watercress, 25g cucumber, 1 beetroot and 3 slices of red onion salad • 1 large wholemeal pitta bread
• 2 oatcakes • 1 orange • 1 pear	• Houmous dip with 2 carrots • 1 orange • 1 kiwi fruit	• 25g tzatziki with 1 carrot stick and 1 celery stick	• 2 rye crispbreads and 40g low-fat cottage cheese
• Diced lamb and chickpea curry: 100g oven-cooked diced lamb, 25g chickpeas, 25g dhal and 150g curry sauce • 50g brown rice	• Turkey stir-fry: 125g turkey breast, 50g bean sprouts, 50g red pepper, 25g chestnuts, 15g soy sauce, 50g mange tout and 1 broccoli spear	• Chilli con carne: 125g pan-fried mince and 150g chilli con carne sauce • 50g rice	• 50g mussels, 75g onions and 12g garlic and 130g tomato sauce • 50g wholemeal pasta
cals 1,605 protein 73g fat 52g carbs 223g fibre 27g	cals 1,389 protein 83g fat 52g carbs 156g fibre 33g	cals 1,472 protein 78g fat 51g carbs 186g fibre 27g	cals 1,513 protein 105g fat 34g carbs 208g fibre 19g

175

Week 8

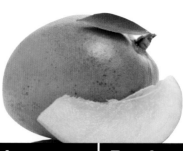

	Monday	Tuesday	Wednesday
Breakfast	• 2 scrambled eggs • 2 grilled tomatoes • 4 mushrooms • 2 wholemeal slices toast • 150ml glass of fresh grapefruit juice	• 2 slices soy-linseed toast • 150g Greek yogurt with 100g blueberries/blackberries • 150ml glass of fresh grapefruit juice	• 140g porridge oats made with skimmed milk • 2 slices wholemeal toast • 150ml glass of fresh grapefruit juice
Mid-morning snacks	• Smoothie made with 250ml soya milk, 1 mango and 1 peach	• 1 apple • 2 rye crispbreads with 1 sliced boiled egg and 5g cress	• 150g low-fat plain yogurt with 100g blackberries
Lunch	• 295g consommé soup with 125g grilled chicken breast and 40g spinach • 1 wholemeal roll	• 125ml kedgeree with 20g watercress • 1 wholegrain roll	• 200g baked potato with small tin of tuna
Mid-afternoon snacks	• 100g blackberries • 2 rye crispbreads with 25g low-fat cottage cheese	• 2 apricots • 1 carrot • 1 celery stick	• 25g taramasalata with 1 celery stick • 1 orange • Handful of strawberries
Dinner	• 150g grilled salmon steak • 80g steamed carrots • 50g mange tout • 150g baked sweet potato	• 100g roast beef • 100g steamed broccoli • 100g green beans • 25g soya beans • 150g roasted sweet potatoes	• Spaghetti Bolognese: 125g pan-fried mince and 250g Bolognese sauce • 50g wholemeal spaghetti
Total daily intake	cals 1,686 **protein** 109g **fat** 67g **carbs** 169g **fibre** 26g	cals 1,483 **protein** 94g **fat** 53g **carbs** 168g **fibre** 31g	cals 1,830 **protein** 107g **fat** 73g **carbs** 198g **fibre** 23g

176

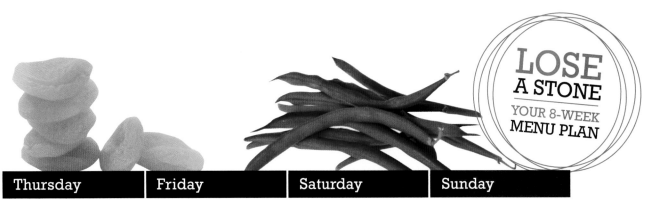

Thursday	Friday	Saturday	Sunday
• 40g sugar-free muesli with 100ml skimmed milk topped with 1 banana • 2 scrambled eggs • 150ml glass of fresh orange juice	• 6 stewed prunes • 30g Bran Flakes with 100ml skimmed milk • 150ml glass of fresh grapefruit juice	• Omelette made with 2 egg whites and 1 whole egg and 50g spinach • 2 slices rye bread • 150ml glass of fresh orange juice	• 1 grilled 120g kipper and 2 tomatoes drizzled with squeeze of lemon juice • 2 slices wholemeal toast • 150ml glass of fresh orange juice
• 150g low-fat yogurt with 100g raspberries	• 50g tzatziki with 2 carrot sticks	• 150g low-fat yogurt with 10g sunflower seeds/flaxseeds and a handful of blackberries • 1 apple • 2 satsumas	• Vegetable juice: 2 celery sticks, 2 carrots, 1 beetroot and pinch of ginger
• 100g reduced sugar and salt baked beans • 2 slices wholemeal toast	• 200g baked potato with 50g sweetcorn and 50g low-fat cottage cheese	• 50g pre-cooked prawns, squeeze of lemon juice and ½ chopped avocado • 2 slices granary bread	• 295g bowl of watercress soup • 1 roast beef baguette: 100g beef, 60g baguette, low-fat spread
• Handful of dried apricots • 25g houmous with 1 carrot and 50g green pepper sticks	• 150g low-fat yogurt • 1 orange • 1 apricot	• 30g tzatziki dip with 1 carrot and 1 celery stick • 1 banana • 1 peach	• 150g fruit yogurt with 2 passion fruits • Small bunch of grapes
• 160g grilled halibut steak • Stir-fry 50g broccoli, 50g green beans, 50g sweetcorn and 25g cashew nuts	• Chicken curry: 125g oven-cooked chicken, 35g okra and 150g curry sauce • 50g brown rice • 1 naan bread	• 150g grilled chicken escalope with 130g tomato sauce • 50g wholemeal spaghetti	• 125g turkey breast steak • 100g steamed broccoli • 25g soya beans • 100g green beans • 200g new potatoes
cals 1,589 **protein** 89g **fat** 63g **carbs** 178g **fibre** 25g	**cals** 1,840 **protein** 82g **fat** 42g **carbs** 301g **fibre** 25g	**cals** 1,655 **protein** 101g **fat** 61g **carbs** 187g **fibre** 25g	**cals** 1,545 **protein** 118g **fat** 40g **carbs** 190g **fibre** 23g

177

Get savvy
Fat of the matter

There are good and bad fats out there, so for perfect health be sure to get the right ones in your diet and you won't go wrong

Fat can be a confusing topic. There are 'good' fats and 'bad' fats. There are fats that make you gain weight and those that help you to lose it. There are foods on the supermarket shelves marketed as low-fat foods, enticing you to select them to help with weight-loss. There are also oily fish products and oily nuts, which are good for a healthy diet. So how do you know what to choose? There are two ways to look at fat if you want to support good health and maintain a desirable bodyweight.

Adding up the calories
Fat is calorific. With just over double the calories in a gram of fat compared to a gram of protein or carbohydrate, you can see why serial dieters throw their arms up in despair and cry 'ban the fat!' The problem with banning fat altogether is that it is essential for bodily functions. Good fats help regulate your blood pressure, heart rate, blood-vessel constriction, blood clotting and your nervous system. In addition, fat carries soluble vitamins (A, E, D and K) from food into the body. Without it we could suffer from deficiencies.

Consider the benefits
The type of fat you select is critical to health and weight maintenance. Good fats include polyunsaturated fats (omega-3 and 6 fats) and monounsaturated fats (omega-9

fats). Omega 3 and 6 fats are vital to maintaining health and are found in nuts, seeds, fish and oils, such as flaxseed, borage and starflower oil. These also reduce inflammation in the body, while providing a stimulatory benefit to the metabolism, and therefore assisting weight-loss.

Good fats are known to reduce bad cholesterol (LDL) and are important in the prevention of heart disease. Aiming for around 20 grams of good fats per day is a great strategy for health support without adding too many calories to the diet.

The bad fat story
Bad fats should be strictly limited in the diet. These include saturated and hydrogenated fats (or trans fats) which are often hidden in fast foods, pastries, cakes, packaged dinners, animal products and some vegetable oils and margarines.

It is difficult to cut these out altogether, but you should limit your intake by eating freshly prepared foods, selecting lean meats and checking food labels for content. A diet high in saturated fat can increase your chances of heart disease, as the body struggles to reduce bad cholesterol levels.

A good way to instantly decrease your intake of hydrogenated fats is to cut out margarine. Try spreading a thin coating of avocado onto breads to create a similar consistency.

In short, don't avoid fat as this can compromise your health. Choosing good fats instead of bad ones and limiting these to 20 grams a day is a great strategy for health and weight management, which will leave you glowing with health inside and out.

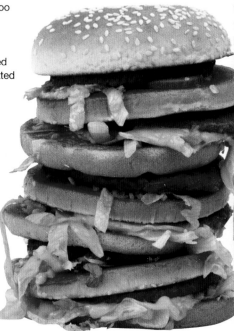